STOP YOUR HUSBAND FROM SNORING

STOP YOUR HUSBAND FROM SNORING

A MEDICALLY PROVEN PROGRAM TO CURE THE NIGHT'S WORST NUISANCE

Derek S. Lipman, M.D.

Rodale Press, Emmaus, Pennsylvania

Printed in the United States of America on acid-free paper ∞

Book design by Diane Ness Shaw
Cover design by Darlene Schneck
Illustrations by Jack Crane and Leslie Flis

If you have any questions or comments concerning this book, please write:
   Rodale Press
   Book Reader Service
   33 East Minor Street
   Emmaus, PA 18098

Library of Congress Cataloging-in-Publication Data

Lipman, Derek S.
   Stop your husband from snoring: a medically proven program to cure the night's worst nuisance/Derek S. Lipman.
      p.   cm.
   Includes bibliographical references.
   ISBN 0-87857-932-X hardcover
   ISBN 0-87857-849-8 paperback
   1. Snoring—Prevention. I. Title.
RA786.3.L56   1990
612.2'1—dc20   90-8284
                                             CIP

Distributed in the book trade by St. Martin's Press

2 4 6 8 10 9 7 5 3 1   hardcover

2 4 6 8 10 9 7 5 3 1   paperback

Notice

This book is intended to provide information and entertainment rather than give specific medical advice or advocate one method of treatment over another.

To accept medical treatment or undergo surgery is a highly personal decision. That decision should be made only after the treating physician has fully explained every aspect of the recommended therapy or procedure, including the options, risks, and possible complications of such treatments.

The author and Rodale Press shall not accept liability or responsibility to any person with respect to loss, injury, or damage caused or alleged to be caused by information contained within this book.

One of my medical school professors was fond of quoting the great physician and teacher, Sir William Osler:

"To study the phenomena of disease without books is to sail an uncharted sea, while to study books without patients is not to go to sea at all."

I dedicate this book to my patients for taking me along on this voyage of discovery.

Contents

Preface

In my 15 years of practice as an ear, nose, and throat specialist, I have consulted with many patients and their partners seeking help for snoring. Sometimes embarrassed, they described to me, in frequently colorful terms, how snoring had disturbed their relationships. Many of these patients spoke of obstructed breathing, choking during the night, and tiredness during the day. They were describing—without realizing the medical significance—a common condition now called (obstructive sleep apnea.)

Until the early 1980s, however, there was little help for the snorer beyond fitting his partner with earplugs. As a physician, it was as frustrating for me to turn a patient away as it was for the patient to leave without getting relief.

Around that time, reports of improved techniques in the diagnosis and treatment of snoring and related sleep-induced breathing disorders began to appear in the medical literature. I became interested in this emerging subject and began attending courses and symposia, visiting sleep disorders clinics, and learning these new techniques from the physicians who had pioneered them. In addition, my interest led me to popular magazine articles on the subject going back to the turn of the century, containing delightful anecdotes about snoring and snorers. In the dusty pages of a 1926 *Ladies' Home Journal*, I discovered the following plea:

> *Experts are sending us mixed messages about snoring. One thing is for certain, there is no simple answer. If you have a solution, write a book. It can't miss. The world is still waiting . . . and snoring.*

Here is my book.

Stop Your Husband from Snoring is not intended as a medical text or a comprehensive review of sleep-related disorders. It is written for snorers and their partners as a way to entertain, to educate, and to encourage them not to take their problem lying down. It is my hope that the information in this book will help many of you, among the millions of snorers, to obtain relief and bring your long-suffering partners out of the spare room and back into the bedroom.

Acknowledgments

I am deeply grateful to the many people whose talent, kindness, and generosity allowed me to bring this book to completion: David Morgan, my agent, whose constant support and encouragement went far beyond the call of duty; editors (now friends) at Rodale Press, Sharon Faelten and Charles Gerras; medical librarians Kathy Rouzie and Susan Westmoreland, Emanuel Hospital and Health Center; Martha Falen, Multnomah County Library; Barbara O'Neill, Patent Specialist, Oregon State Library, Salem; Tom Stave, Documents Department, University of Oregon Library, Eugene; reference librarians, Lake Oswego (Oregon) Public Library; Lucy Seger, R.PSG.T., The Association of Polysomnographic Technologists; Frank Adams, Executive Director, American Sleep Disorders Foundation; Department of Medical Photography, St. Vincent Hospital and Medical Center; Jack L. Gluckman, M.D., Department of Otolaryngology and Maxillofacial Surgery, College of Medicine, University of Cincinnati; Louis S. Libby, M.D., Director of the Sleep Disorders Laboratory, Providence Medical Center, Portland; F. Blair Simmons, M.D., Division of Otolaryngology—Head and Neck Surgery, Stanford University Medical Center; Mary Kay Norby, Sleep Care, Inc.; Kathleen Spiekerman and Barbara Petrick, R.N., Sleep Physiology Services; Thomas A. Meade, D.D.S.; Edward R. Clements, Mountain Medical Equipment, Inc.; Marty Douglass, Respironics, Inc.;

Gerald B. Rich, M.D., Director, Pacific Northwest Sleep/ Wake Disorders Program, Good Samaritan Hospital and Medical Center, Portland; American Sleep Disorders Association; Instructors of the American Academy of Otolaryngology—Head and Neck Surgery, too numerous to mention, whose superb presentations and informal discussions provided so much valuable information; transcriptionists Ruth Perrigo and Chris Ragel; William Taylor, Senior Systems Consultant, Wang Laboratories, Portland; G. Nino-Murcia, M.D., Director, Sleep Disorders Clinic, Stanford University; Alfred J. Schroeder, M.D.; Kathy Hanlon Frazier, who oversees my practice with a sunny nature and dazzling efficiency; and to my family, whose support and understanding allowed me to lead a cloistered existence while trying to meet the deadline. I will make it up to them.

A Handy Guide to Stopping Your Husband's Snoring—From A to Zzzz

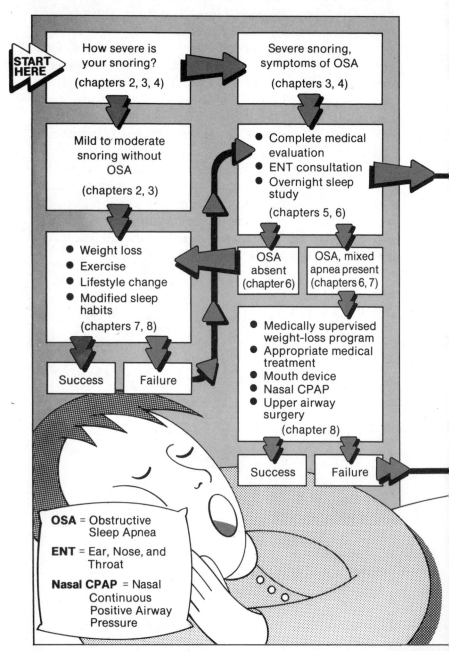

START HERE

How severe is your snoring?

(chapters 2, 3, 4)

Severe snoring, symptoms of OSA

(chapters 3, 4)

Mild to moderate snoring without OSA

(chapters 2, 3)

- Complete medical evaluation
- ENT consultation
- Overnight sleep study

(chapters 5, 6)

- Weight loss
- Exercise
- Lifestyle change
- Modified sleep habits

(chapters 7, 8)

OSA absent (chapter 6)

OSA, mixed apnea present (chapters 6, 7)

- Medically supervised weight-loss program
- Appropriate medical treatment
- Mouth device
- Nasal CPAP
- Upper airway surgery

(chapter 8)

Success

Failure

Success

Failure

OSA = Obstructive Sleep Apnea

ENT = Ear, Nose, and Throat

Nasal CPAP = Nasal Continuous Positive Airway Pressure

Here is a graphic overview of the stages of snoring, its physical effects, and the resources this book offers as you struggle to return to the peaceful nights and pleasant dreams you once enjoyed.

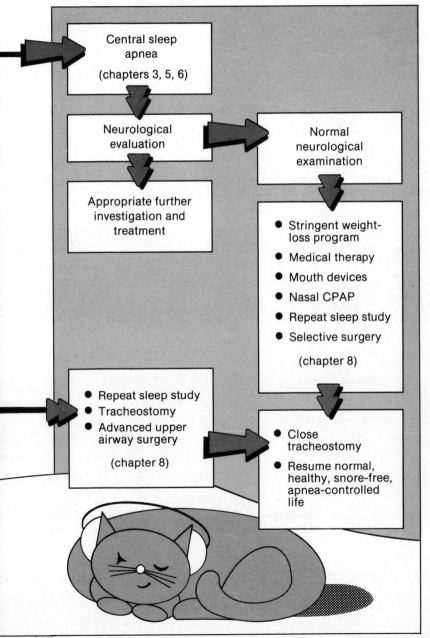

CHAPTER 1

Is There
a Snorer
in the House?

S leep.
Poets have praised it as the ultimate symbol for rest
and quietude. Longfellow referred to it as "night's repose," Shakespeare called it "nature's soft nurse," and
Keats exulted "O magic sleep! O comfortable bird/That
broodest o'er the troubled sea of mind/Till it is hushed
and smooth."

But few of us are poets, and for many, sleep is far from
"magic" and often quite far from "hushed and smooth."
As an anxious wife wrote to popular columnist Abigail
Van Buren:

> Dear Abby:
> I am desperately trying to find a cure for my
> husband's snoring. After being married for 27 years,
> I am convinced there is no cure other than killing
> him, which is illegal in our country.

1

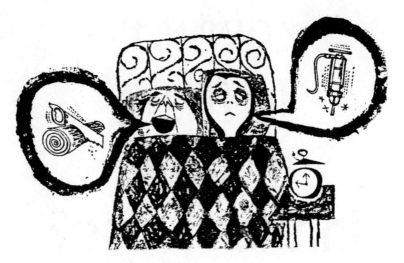

He may be just "sawing wood," but his snores nearly equal the sound level of a jackhammer.

Snoring has been with us since time began. It is not difficult to imagine our prehistoric ancestors sleeping in their caves, rumbling and snorting in the flickering firelight. In fact, according to one theory, present-day snorers are simply reenacting the primitive instinct of making loud noises at night to protect their sleeping womenfolk. Many men may cite this theory as proof of their manly devotion, saying "I'm just keeping the woolly mammoths away from you, Dear." But few women today seem willing to buy it!

Over 40 million Americans snore. For some, snoring is no more than an occasional and innocuous habit. But for countless wives it represents an unending nightly disturbance that turns what Milton called the "kindly dew of sleep" into a disruptive, nerve-racking experience. No doubt this is what philosopher/author Anthony Burgess had in mind when he wrote his famous epigram: "Laugh and the world laughs with you; snore and you sleep alone."

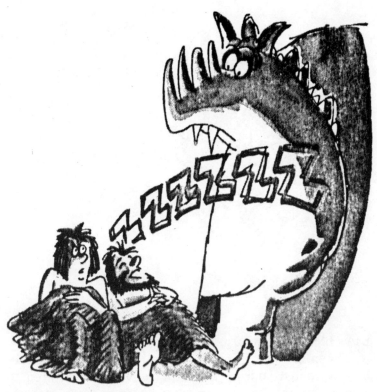

Snorers Are Immune to the Noise

Regarded as everything from a bother to a joke, the snorer has been looked upon as a whimsical oddity—a kind of misfit whose trumpetings make him an ideal subject for humorists. Mark Twain devoted an entire essay to the subject, marveling that the snorer could somehow manage to sleep blissfully, while those around him had to cover their ears. "There ain't no way to find out," he moaned, "why a snorer can't hear himself snore." And later, Twain's immortal Huckleberry Finn said of his father in awe: "Pap used to sleep . . . with the hogs, but

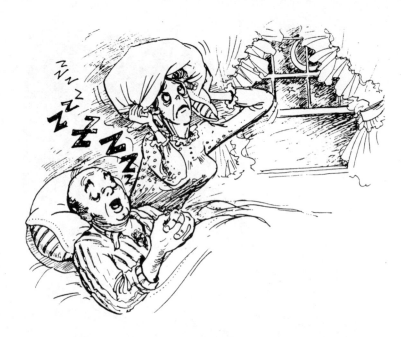

Laws bless you, he just lifts things when he snores."

Even in the military, where all things male are cele-brated, robust snoring is neither envied nor aspired to. The illustrious Roman statesman Marcus Cato withered one of his generals by declaring, "His snore is louder than his battle cry."

Some might say that America was settled as the roundabout result of a snore. John Smith, a young English commander in charge of a 150-horse unit (assigned to drive the Turks from Hungary), found his way to Po-cahontas and into American history because of a sentry who slept, snoring at his post. Drawn by the sound of the sentry's extraordinary sawing, a passing army of Tartars discovered Smith's sleeping camp and attacked immedi-ately. In the massacre that followed, Smith was captured and sold as a slave in Constantinople. He escaped and walked hundreds of miles across Europe, finally arriving back in England. There, using new maps and data gathered as he worked his way home, he organized an expedition for the New World land of Virginia. Good fortune led him to befriend Pocahontas, the Indian chief's daughter, who saved him from beheading. And the rest, as they say, is history.

Perhaps the most celebrated snorer to wear the uniform of his country was Private Tony Rodriguez, a United States M.P. stationed in London, England, during World War II. A barracks' mate, who evidently suffered through many a sleepless night, finally wrote these program notes about Tony's virtuoso performance:

> *The first movement is pastoral. Then . . . the violas and double basses enter vigorously. The second movement introduces the sounds of war. Fighter planes rise in a screeching spiral to give battle to a bomber formation. The intermingled aircraft fire all their guns and cannons, and the bombers release heavy salvos of high-explosive bombs.*
>
> *Tony shifts in his sleep, and the third movement begins, more soul-searing than the second. A man is drowning in a heavy storm at sea. We hear the mountainous crash of the waves, the screams of the lost man, the mournful bellows of a whistling buoy, and the peals of angry thunder. Then comes the unbearable crash of the massed kettledrums. A shoe hits Tony. The symphony is over.*

The records show that Rodriguez's commanding officer saved the morale of the company by ordering a special hut built for him. Presumably Tony continued to develop his musical gifts while sleeping alone.

Snoring respects neither social nor economic boundaries. Numerous presidents of the United States are said to have been impressive snorers, including Washington, both Adamses, Lincoln, Taft, and Franklin Delano Roosevelt. And, although it sullies his image a bit, the famed British lady's man, Beau Brummell, was known as a prodigious snorer, as were Churchill and Mussolini.

Duel of the Decibels

Some of the truly outrageous snorers managed to capitalize on their vice. David Bishop, reputed to be the champion snorer of the great state of Arizona, was challenged by Texan Steve Hawkins to a Snore-Down. The bet was $10,000. The two men checked into adjoining rooms at a local hotel to do their stuff for the judges (the town undertaker and a magistrate), who stood outside the bedroom doors to evaluate the thunder. But the contest was declared a draw. A second bout was scheduled, but before it began, the judges were approached by a white-haired old man, a stranger in town, who wore ill-fitting clothes and spoke with a heavy German accent. He introduced himself as the famous Professor August von Dusenberg, inventor of the phonometer, a scientific sound-measuring machine. The professor volunteered the use of his invention as a foolproof way to decide the winner. His offer was gratefully accepted.

When the snoring began that evening, the professor pressed the button to start his machine. Fascinated, the judges watched as a series of staccato snorts advanced the indicator closer and closer to the highest mark. Suddenly, there was a mighty roar of a snore and something snapped in the machine. The indicator shot back to zero and stayed there. And that's where the story ends. Bishop's and Hawkins's snoring had broken the machine! No clear winner ever emerged in that contest. Nor was a stronger phonometer ever invented.

The true snoring champion of the world is Melvin Switzer, according to the *Guinness Book of World Records*. Using recording equipment provided by the local Noise Abatement Society, mighty Mel outblasted his competitors during the early morning hours in a contest held at Hever Castle in Kent, England, on June 28, 1984. He proudly took first place with a snore score of 87.5 decibels—the equivalent of a motorcycle revving up at close quarters. (Note: Switzer's wife is deaf in one ear.)

You're Not Dreaming—It's Loud!

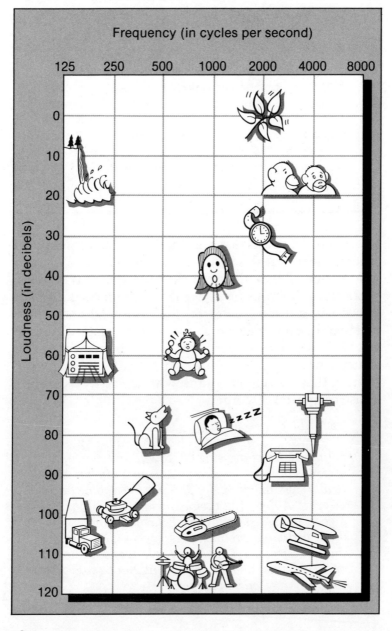

Silent Night

"It blasts the silence of the night like an open-throttled Mack truck warming into an uphill climb. It crashes through the central nervous system like a jackhammer; it whines like a chain saw wasting a forest. It is punctuated by uneven arrhythmic snorts—the triumphant blurt of water buffalo."
Marcia Cohen, *Ladies' Home Journal*, October, 1976.

It's no surprise that snoring has turned roommates into enemies, cut short the budding relationship of many a young couple, and blasted the bliss out of the honeymoon for numerous newlyweds. Once married, the language wives use to report on their husband's snoring is alternately anguished, desperate, bitter, resigned, or wistful. This letter represents many that distressed and exhausted wives write to columnist Abigail Van Buren, suggesting that snoring may rank with infidelity as a prime cause of marital discord:

Dear Abby:

I woke up at three o'clock this morning, wondering who was mowing our lawn. Another time, I dreamed a tugboat was stuck in our bedroom, frantically signaling for help. This has been going on for 15 years, Abby. I can't remember the last time I had a good night's sleep. When I threaten to go to another bedroom, my husband says he didn't marry me to sleep alone. I have begged him to see a doctor or try remedies I have heard about. But he won't. He says I snore. Can you help me?

Frantic in Fresno

The Great International Noise Neutralizer

Even in Bavaria, snoring is not exactly *The Sound of Music*. So be prepared to declare peace wherever you travel. Just look signora or madame straight in the eye and demand: "Stop Your Husband from Snoring!"

Here's how to be sure you're understood. When you want to:

Relax in Rome, rage:	*"Impedisci a tuo marito di russare!"*
Pass a pleasant night in Paris, plead:	*"¡Empêcher votre mari de ronfler!"*
Ease the pain in Spain, complain:	*"¡No dejes que tu marido ronque!"*
Cut the cacophony in Copenhagen, command:	*"Stop din mands snorken!"*
Head off a Hungarian rhapsody, rasp:	*"Hogyan érjük el, hogy férjünk ne horkoljon!"*
Get some zzzzs in Zambia, say:	*"Lesha minkonono ya mulume woobe!"*

More than 150,000 replies poured in. Some readers offered sympathy; others advice. Over 90 percent moved to another bedroom as soon as one became available.

Sprinkled with wisdom and imagination, their letters portrayed wives whom fate had left with the choice of either lying awake in the darkness while the walls around them shook, or taking a lonely trip down the hall to the spare bedroom. Their marriages, once the stuff of dreams, had turned into nightmares.

The Trouble with George

Perhaps the most celebrated letter about snoring in matrimony came not from a woman but from a man. In April 1915, George Little of Pittsburgh, Pennsylvania, wrote to the *Ladies' Home Journal* asking readers for advice on how to stop his disruptive habit. Readers' replies poured in from all over the country with recommendations, information, and sympathy. So numerous were the responses that the *Journal* started a column that ran for a year, entitled "How Can 'George' Stop Snoring?" These were among the answers that came in:

> *I never used to snore until my hair began to fall out, and the balder I got the louder I snored . . . . Finally my wife . . . brought from town one day a slumber cap, which I have worn ever since—at night, of course—and I have ceased to snore. You see, my hair was so thin that I caught cold every night, and stuffing up, would snore.*

Signed: **Atlanta**

> *Do you realize that Indians never snore? I have slept many a night in their teepees and never a sound. The secret of it is that Indian children are always taught to sleep with their mouth closed so as to prevent throat troubles. Here is a hint for mothers if we are to prevent another generation of snorers.*

Signed: **Mrs. D. R.**

> *As snoring comes from within, we must look for the cause within. If a man were truly unselfish and refined, he would not snore. He would be the same within as without and the same asleep as awake. What we are within is bound to come out. Therefore,*

the only permanent cure for snoring is to be wholly unselfish in every thought, and natural refinement will come; and then—men will not snore.

Signed: **Helen Howard**

Eventually, the unending flood of letters from thousands of anxious readers forced the editors of the *Journal* to cry, "Enough! If Mr. Little hasn't enough 'cures' by this time, the *Journal* fears he is hopeless!"

Too bad George didn't see this ad running in the newspapers of the day:

I Can Absolutely Cure Snoring

By a simple remedy that all physicians will unqualifiedly endorse. No medicine, no mechanical contrivances; just a simple rule, which followed, does away with even the most aggravated cases of snoring.

Send $1 to _____

Understandably excited, many snorers quickly sent in their dollar and just as quickly received this printed response:

An Absolute Cure
for Snoring
Don't Go to Sleep

While such stories showed that snoring could bring out the larceny in us, other accounts indicate that snoring gave rise to even more drastic "cures." In Budapest, in 1923, a woman was arrested for murder when she admitted that she could no longer tolerate her husband's snoring and finally pulled out a pistol and killed him. And as recently as 1989, in Winthrop, Massachusetts, a man stood trial for allegedly strangling his elderly hospital roommate because the victim's snoring kept him awake all night.

John Wesley Hardin, the fabled gunfighter, became incensed by the snoring of a man in the room next to his in the American House Hotel in Abilene, Texas. Not one to waste time with his feelings, Hardin began firing his gun through the bedroom wall. The first bullet awoke the stranger; the second one killed him. Years later, Hardin tried to set the record straight. "They tell lots of lies about me," he complained. "They say I killed six or seven men for snoring. Well, it ain't true, I only killed one." Regardless of the number, Hardin certainly diminished the population of snorers in Texas. But he left plenty behind. Nobody knows how many serious snorers rattle the shutters every night.

Snorers: Wake Up and Be Counted!

Virtually all of us snore now and then. Much of it is mild or occasional snoring—as when a man comes home

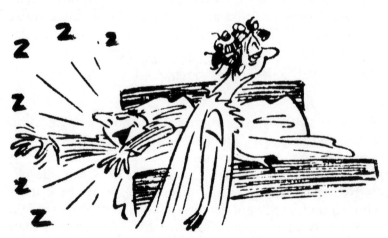

Snore—and you may soon snore alone!

from a tiring day, falls asleep, and begins to saw away. Given a poke in the ribs, he changes position, and his snoring stops.

Generally, researchers don't include this type of snoring in any statistical study. Additionally, even truly serious snorers do not readily admit to the habit—so studies of its prevalence are all the more difficult and imprecise. In fact, it wasn't until 1968 when Marcus Boulware, Ph.D., a speech pathologist, director of the Speech and Hearing Program at Florida A. & M. University in Tallahassee, and a pioneer snore therapist as well, made a significant attempt to research the incidence of snoring. Upon questioning 50 state health departments for information on snoring statistics, he found that there were none. A man whose snoring had nearly ended his own marriage, Dr. Boulware asked for and received a $100,000 research grant from the National Institutes of Health to find a cure for snoring. His initiative must have inspired other researchers throughout the world to delve into the mysteries of snoring.

In 1978 a team of medical researchers led by Elio Lugaresi, M.D., conducted a study of the inhabitants of San Marino, an independent republic of 20,000 people in northern Italy. From a questionnaire on snoring and sleep disturbances, Dr. Lugaresi determined that 20 percent of all the people who responded snored regularly, that twice as many males as females admitted to snoring, and that snoring in men and women appeared to increase with age. Between the ages of 30 to 35, 20 percent of males and 5 percent of females snored regularly. From ages 60 to 65, however, 60 percent of the men reported snoring and so did 40 percent of the women.

In a 1983 investigation done in Toronto on the prevalence of snoring, questionnaires were given to 254 consecutive patients attending a family practice clinic in the city and 25 consecutive patients in a clinic in a rural community in northern Ontario. Despite the environmental and geographic differences, the results in each group were so similar that they were not separated in the analysis.

- 86 percent of the women said their husband snored.
- 52 percent of the women said they were troubled by their husband's snoring.
- 57 percent of the men said their wife snored.
- 15 percent of the men said that they were troubled by their wife's snoring.
- The majority of snorers were male, outnumbering the females 9 to 1.

But helpful as these findings are, more studies must be conducted before we can get an accurate idea about the universality of this habit. In the meantime, the expanding number of sleep disorders centers and greater public and medical awareness of snoring are contributing to a deeper, more sophisticated body of literature on the subject.

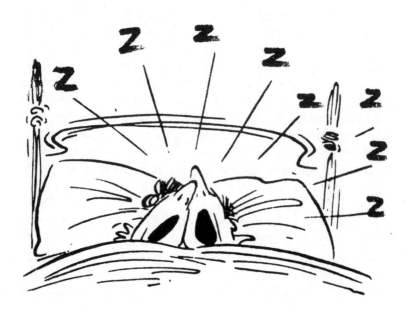

Some **Good** Snoring Stories

Before we explore these findings, let's return to our history of snoring to demonstrate that snoring does indeed have a positive side.

Ormund Powers could have been the first columnist to suggest that snoring may be a source of comfort and reassurance. "Snoring is the magic of sleep," he wrote in the *Orlando Sentinel-Star.* "It causes far less difficulties among married couples than the absence of snoring brought about when the snorer is not there." Echoing this sentiment was a letter to columnist Abigail Van Buren from a widow, lamenting that to her, snoring would be the sweetest sound this side of heaven. Perhaps it was such sentiments that led to immortalizing the charm of the snore by naming an inn I came across near Victoria, British Columbia: Great-Snoring-On-Sea.

And finally, this delightful short story "The Snoring Beauty," by Anne Douglas Sedgwick, published many years ago in *Harper's Magazine:*

> *Launcelot Mainwaring was clearly falling head over heels in love with a beautiful young lady, Elizabeth Thayer, while vacationing in Paris, where they were both staying in the same hotel near the Champs Elysees.*
>
> *After being introduced by mutual friends, Mainwaring invited Ms. Thayer to attend a performance of the opera* Romeo and Juliet. *By the end of the second act, he was hopelessly in love with her.*
>
> *Returning to the hotel, they retired to their adjacent rooms, whereupon Mainwaring was suddenly awakened by the deafening sound of snoring coming from the next room where his loved one slept.*
>
> *After enduring three nights of this fearsome din, Mainwaring took his beloved aside, confessed his undying love, and, with unabashed candor, told her of her terrible snoring. Elizabeth, upon hearing this, dropped into a nearby chair, shaking with*

*laughter. When she could finally control herself, she
confided to Mainwaring that the source of the snoring was her little dog Toto. "But," she added, "you
are a perfect hero. How you must have suffered these
nights. I think," she said, her eyes aglow with pas-
sion for her new suitor, "you are a man to be
adored."*

A Brighter Future

Those who have attempted to go beyond folk remedies and seek professional help have followed further on
the path of frustration. Until recently, medical men were
sadly lacking in a scientific approach to this subject, and
they had little in the way of remedies to offer the snoring
patient.

As recently as 20 years ago, for example, the grim
prognosis for snorers was summed up by the editor of the
British Medical Association's popular monthly *Family
Doctor:* "I'm not hopeful about a cure for snoring," he
wrote. "It is unlikely that anyone will come up with
anything dramatic or sensational."

Today however, snoring has graduated from being
regarded as a hopeless nightly nuisance to the level of a
legitimate medical problem—as respectable a symptom
as back pain or headache. Researchers and clinicians have
finally isolated the underlying causes of snoring and are
now discovering a variety of realistic treatments for it.
These can bring gratifying results to both snorers and
snorees.

CHAPTER 2

Searching for the Cause

In the first chapter we looked at snoring in the superficial way people usually do—as a stressful nuisance—funny to some and infuriating to others. But to understand it fully, we need to know what the term "snoring" really means. Unfortunately, it is easier to discover the causes of snoring than it is to define it.

Webster's New International Dictionary defines snoring as "breathing during sleep with a rough, hoarse noise due to vibration of the uvula and soft palate." However, most ear, nose, and throat specialists subscribe to the definition that snoring is "any resonant noise produced in the upper respiratory tract during sleep." But the descriptions of that "resonant noise" vary widely, from snorting, rasping, choking, and gasping, to rattling, sawing, rumbling, and hissing. Obviously, we can describe snoring in myriad ways, just as Eskimos have a hundred different words for snow, and each is correct, depending

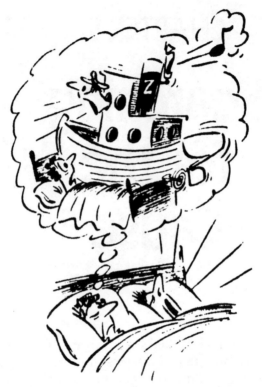

A classic among the many ways wives have found to describe their mate's snoring: "I dreamed a tugboat was stuck in our bedroom, frantically signaling for help."

on our individual experience. Perhaps Mark Twain put it best when he wrote that snoring is "sleeping out loud."

What's Your Snore Level?

To obtain a more precise frame of reference, physicians have developed an objective classification system for the degree of noise produced by snoring.

Mild: Occasional snoring, usually while the sleeper

is lying on his back and is overtired or has drunk too much alcohol or eaten too much food.

Moderate: Frequent snoring that occurs in all body positions.

Severe: Very loud snoring that continues throughout the night in all body positions and can be heard from one or two rooms away.

Heroic: Extremely loud snoring that can be heard from three or four rooms away or throughout the entire house.

Though they are far from exact, these descriptions do allow us to explore the causes of snoring by associating it with two distinct facts: (1) The sound of snoring is produced in the upper respiratory tract, and (2) snoring occurs during sleep.

Summer Snoring Is the Loudest

Each year, the coming of summer transforms many bedrooms into noisy torture chambers, according to modern snore lore. The reason: Scientists have shown that men snore louder and longer during the shorter nights of summer than they do in winter, and the fault lies with the sun. Longer days mean more chance to absorb ultraviolet rays from the sun, which produces more relaxation at bedtime. The more relaxed, the more vigorous the snoring.

Solving Some Puzzles of Snoring

Everyone knows that snoring occurs during sleep. But the questions that have always mystified the partners of snorers and, until recently, physicians as well, are these: Why does snoring occur *only* during sleep? And why are we more likely to snore when we sleep on our back than on our stomach? Why, in other words, don't we snore standing up? Or when we're awake?

Scientific research into sleep didn't begin until late in the nineteenth century, when the electrical activity of the brains of rabbits, cats, and monkeys was recorded. Then, many years later in 1929, a German psychiatrist, Hans Berger, M.D., recorded human electrical brain activity and coined the term *electroencephalogram (EEG)* for this process. His work prepared the way for examining various brain functions—normal activities such as sleep, as well as numerous disorders of the brain and nervous system.

But Dr. Berger's findings about the electrical activity of the brain during sleep were virtually ignored for nearly a decade. Then, in 1937, a team of independent researchers confirmed and advanced his findings through their all-night sleep studies, which demonstrated alternating stages in sleep, distinguished by the brain's varying electrical patterns during each stage. In 1953, researchers at the University of Chicago discovered the rapid eye movement (REM) stage of sleep, named for the rapid eye movements that characterized it. Presumably REM sleep eluded earlier researchers because it looked so much like an awake period when recorded on an EEG printout. These researchers thought that their subjects had simply awakened during the night, when, in fact (and this was the most exciting understanding to come from the discovery of REM sleep), they were *dreaming*. Today, sleep is spoken of as passing through two distinct phases: REM sleep and non-REM (NREM) sleep.

We Sleep in Stages

A closer look at REM and NREM sleep brings us to our first answer concerning questions about the causes of snoring and its curious association with sleep.

Stage 1—NREM sleep: A transitional stage between wakefulness and sleep, usually lasting 5 to 10 minutes. Breathing becomes slow and regular, the heart rate decreases, and we see slow, rolling eye movements. This stage accounts for 5 to 10 percent of a person's total sleep time.

Stage 2—NREM sleep: A deeper stage of sleep, where fragmented thoughts and images pass through the mind. Eye movements usually disappear, muscles relax, and there is very little body movement. This stage predominates in adults, representing about 50 percent of total sleep time.

Stage 3—NREM sleep: Further deepening of sleep with additional slowing of heart and breathing rates. The body's temperature falls; eye movements are absent. This phase comprises approximately 25 percent of the total sleep time in children and adolescents, declines slightly in young adults, and decreases dramatically in middle age and older years.

Stage 4—NREM sleep: The deepest phase of sleep. Arousal in this stage is the most difficult. Typically, sleepwalking and bedwetting occur at this time. Stage 4 usually occurs only during the first third of the night, after which NREM sleep does not progress beyond stage 3. Because these two phases of sleep are so similar, researchers have frequently described them in combination. Together they comprise 10 to 20 percent of our total sleep time, diminishing with age.

The NREM stages of our sleep cycle are notable for their physiological rest and quiet. Eye movements are infrequent, heart and respiratory rates are reduced, and the body is still. When awakened from NREM sleep, people commonly describe vague fragmented thoughts, scenes, or images.

REM sleep: After about 90 minutes of NREM sleep, the first period of REM sleep begins. Initially lasting a few minutes, the REM phase increases to 15 to 20 minutes' duration as sleep progresses.

This phase is distinguished from other sleep stages by a dramatic decrease in muscle tone. The skeletal muscles of the neck, arms, and legs are essentially paralyzed. Breathing becomes irregular, the heart rate increases, and the eyes display rapid, darting movements. The soft tissues of the upper airway, including the tongue, soft palate, and uvula, are completely relaxed. During this phase, the brain's oxygen consumption increases. Sweating, shivering, and other body temperature-regulatory mechanisms are usually absent during REM sleep. In males, REM sleep is associated with penile erection.

A Busy Time for Your Brain

REM sleep is the sleep stage of dreaming, typified by vivid, active dreams, consisting of complex symbols and images. Over 70 percent of adults awakened during REM sleep report dreaming. This stage constitutes about 20 percent of the total sleep time for an adult.

The cycle of sleep stages continues throughout the night as we alternate between NREM and REM sleep. Most commonly, the NREM stages develop during the first third of the sleep period, and REM sleep and stage 2 NREM sleep predominate during the last third. REM sleep usually enters the cycle as we move from stage 3 or 4 NREM sleep back to stage 2, and the whole cycle repeats itself in time periods that can range from 70 to 120 minutes. As you would expect, those who require a greater amount of sleep spend more time in REM sleep, but even

Riding the Sleep-Wake Cycle

We know that sleep provides restoration for our body as well as our mind. And all living creatures have cycles of alternating activity and rest. For some animals, the cycle is determined by environmental changes such as the fluctuation of the tides; for others, a change in seasons may signal the switch from activity to hibernation. In man, the sleep-wake cycle occurs over a period of approximately 24 hours (25 hours to be exact), apparently governed by an internal clock as well as outside changes such as darkness or light. This pattern, called circadian (around the day) rhythm, is established in infants after three or four months and continues throughout life.

Does our internal clock run down with age? No one knows. But age does seem to reset it. The elderly tend to go to bed earlier than young people, wake up earlier, and generally have a shorter total sleep time.

Lack of sleep or sudden changes in the sleep-wake cycle can, and does, produce alterations in mood, performance, and vigilance. These disturbances can vary in severity, depending upon the number of hours shifted, the frequency of the work shifts, and the amount of time allowed for new normal sleep-wake cycles to develop. Similar sleep disturbances are experienced by air travelers, whose jet lag is a result of disrupted body rhythms due to changing time zones.

those who require very little sleep go through the customary cycle.

Theories abound as to how and why we use REM
sleep and its associated dream state to reenact and process
experiences we have had during wakefulness. Under ideal
conditions of sleep our bodies are virtually at rest and so
they permit the greatest attention to mental (psychological) activity. But studies also show that REM sleep occurs
in unborn babies. Obviously, more research must be conducted before we can grasp the full meaning and value of
REM sleep.

What we do know, however, is that the sleep cycle is
directly related to snoring, and for evidence of that we
need to correlate sleep and the anatomical structures that
produce the snores.

The Source of the Noise

Snoring originates in those parts of your upper air
passages called the collapsible part of the throat, or the
collapsible airway. By collapsible, we mean that the soft
tissues of this region have no rigid framework or support.
They include the soft palate, uvula, tonsils, tissues
around the tonsils (called tonsillar pillars), the base of the
tongue, and the back and sidewalls of the throat.

The sounds are produced in the collapsible airway
through vibrations of the soft tissues located there. These
vibrations occur because of turbulence in the airway of
the sleeper as he breathes through his nose or mouth,
producing a flutter-valve effect in the soft tissues that can
be likened to wind rattling a loose windowpane, or a flag
snapping back and forth in a stiff breeze. Ironically,
sleep—that state of quiet repose and relaxation—actually
contributes to the production of snoring by creating the
greatest amount of slack in the body's structural material
(muscles and tissues) and leaving them susceptible to this
flutter effect when conditions are right.

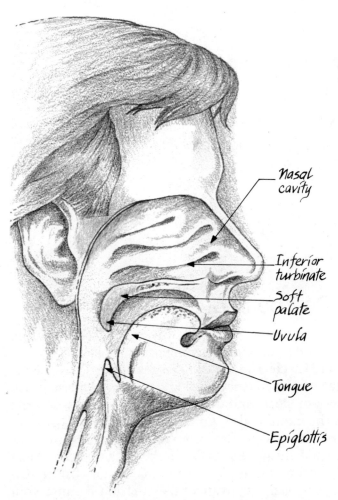

nasal
cavity

Inferior
turbinate

Soft
palate

Uvula

Tongue

Epiglottis

Side view of the nose and throat.

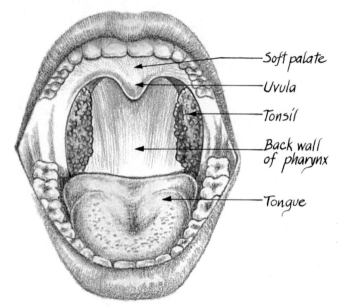

Soft palate

Uvula

Tonsil

Back wall of pharynx

Tongue

View of the mouth and upper throat.

Why Do You Snore?

With that information, the various causes of snoring and its association with sleeping become clear.

Poor Muscle Tone in the Tissues of the Throat: During sleep, the degree of muscle relaxation increases with the depth of sleep, and the more relaxed the tissues, the greater the likelihood of vibration and the sounds of snoring. As we have seen, maximum muscle relaxation occurs during REM sleep—especially in the neck muscles. Most snoring occurs, therefore, during this period of sleep. Lying on your back aggravates this situation because your tongue customarily falls backward into your upper airway due to the relaxed muscles there, augmented by the pull of gravity. This narrows the opening of your airway, forcing greater air flow over the already relaxed tissues.

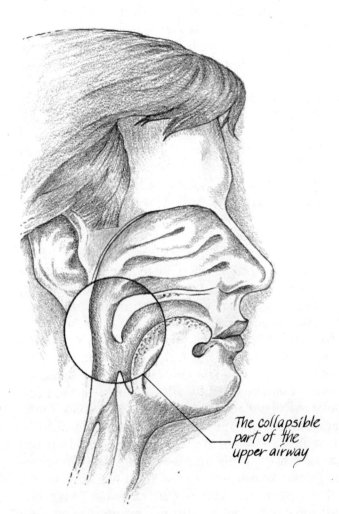

The collapsible
part of the
upper airway

The upper breathing passages.

Muscle tone in the tissues of the throat also slackens with age. (Just think of the sagging skin under an older person's chin.) As our upper airway tissues become more floppy and less resilient with age, even in our waking state, it isn't surprising that snoring increases significantly as people get older.

Snoring and Obesity: Although the exact mechanisms by which obesity causes or aggravates snoring are unclear, we do know that the thick neck structures so frequently seen in overweight people tend to narrow the air passages. Moreover these individuals often have flabby tissues, with poor muscle tone, from lack of exercise.

Increased Bulk in the Soft Tissues of the Throat: Large tonsils or adenoids narrow the air passage by taking up space, and that encourages snoring. The bulky neck tissues in some heavyset individuals have a similar effect. A long uvula and soft palate also reduce the size of a person's airway and increase the flutter-valve effect, which contributes to the sound of snoring. Certain anatomical factors, such as a receding chin, can cause the tongue to protrude backward and aggravate the normal falling-back effect that already has occurred during sleep. An underactive thyroid or Down's syndrome, for example, are often characterized by a large tongue which further blocks the upper airway during sleep.

Drugs, Fatigue, and Smoking: Tranquilizers, antihistamines, or alcohol, taken in excess and prior to sleep, can aggravate snoring by deepening a person's sleep and causing even greater than normal relaxation of upper airway tissues. Overeating or overworking can also exaggerate the conditions that lead to snoring by increasing your exhaustion, resulting in over-relaxation of upper airway tissues. Smoking, though not a direct cause of snoring, contributes to it by causing the mucous membranes in the throat to swell and restrict the air passages.

Aside from these factors, any obstruction in your nasal passages can contribute to snoring when that nasal

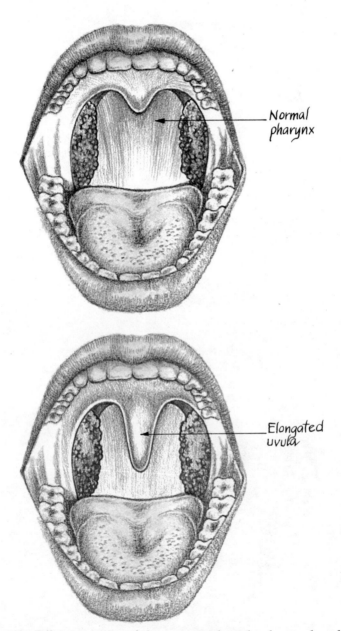

Normal
pharynx

Elongated
uvula

Note the difference in size of these two uvulas: The elongated uvula narrows the air passage, contributing to snoring.

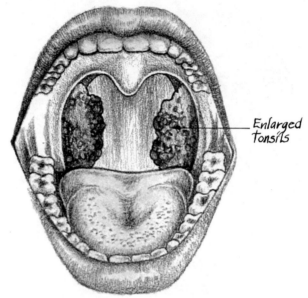

View of obstructive tonsils.

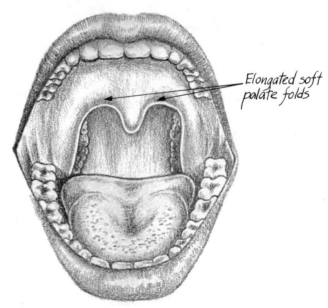

View of obstructive soft palate folds.

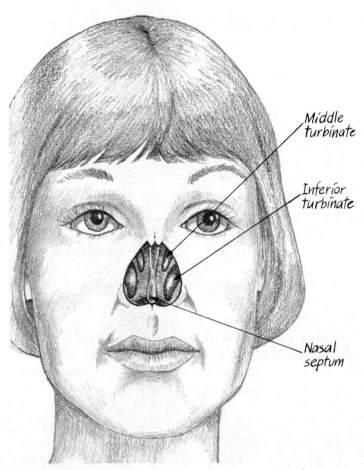

Middle turbinate

Inferior turbinate

Nasal septum

The normal nose structure.

obstruction is coupled with the changes you undergo during sleep. So why don't we simply work around the nasal obstruction by breathing through our mouth?

Why We Persist in Nasal Breathing

First, even though you breathe through your mouth as well as through your nose, there seems to be some

instinctive desire to breathe through the nose anyway—
even when the nostrils are severely obstructed. For example, think of the discomfort you go through with acute
nasal congestion from the flu or a cold. You can breathe
perfectly well through your mouth during these times,
yet you frantically seek out an effective nasal decongestant. One reason for this curious phenomenon is that you
actually increase the work of breathing when you breathe
through your mouth, bringing on physical fatigue as well
as psychological anxiety.

Second, studies show that resistance in the oral airway is actually greater than resistance in the nasal airway
when we are asleep lying down. During sleep, the nasal
airway seems to be the body's preferred route for
breathing, compared with the path of higher resistance
that oral breathing offers. To understand this, we have to
return to our discussion of the anatomical changes that
occur during the stages of sleep.

During normal sleep, the firmness of your throat
muscles slackens, the airway narrows, and increased resistance to inspiration follows—because the passageway
through which your breath must pass is reduced. This
normal collapse of your throat tissues as the muscles
relax, restricts the space in your upper airway and brings
the soft tissues more directly into the path of your breath.

Breathing-in power (we call this inspiratory pressure)
must increase in order to counteract this natural narrowing of the upper airway during sleep. As the sleeper's
effort to breathe increases, greater pressure is exerted on
the soft tissues of the pharynx, which are pulled inward,
and as a result, they may begin fluttering. This produces
snoring.

If the nose is completely blocked, the sleeper is required to breathe entirely through his mouth. This narrows the air passage even more, as air passing into the
throat directly from the mouth produces a negative pres-

sure in the back of the throat by sucking in the soft tissues of the collapsible airway.

You can re-create this effect while awake by lying down, and, with your mouth closed, breathing slowly and deeply through your nose. If there's no obstruction, the air should pass through effortlessly. Now, hold your nose closed and breathe slowly and deeply through your mouth. You should be more aware of air passing over your collapsible tissues and you should also feel these tissues being pulled in slightly as the air creates a vacuum. Current research suggests that the firm bone and cartilage structures that support the nasal airway prevent this vacuum effect from occurring when you breathe through your nose.

Some Common Nasal Causes of Snoring

If nasal obstruction causes disturbances in normal, wakeful breathing, then it's not surprising that such obstruction complicates nighttime breathing and contributes to snoring. Just knowing the possible causes of nasal obstruction is of great value in determining whether or not you snore and where you might begin to look for factors that bring it on. For example, hay fever might contribute to snoring without ever being spotted as the culprit. If the sufferer is lean and fit and is a nondrinker and/or a nonsmoker, he might futilely resign himself to his snoring as some quirk of nature and never realize that it's due to his seasonal allergy.

Similarly, a pregnant woman might become confused and embarrassed when she suddenly begins snoring. If she realizes that nasal congestion is a common occurrence in the early stages of pregnancy, and may be the reason she breathes in through her mouth, she will be more at ease.

Here are some of the many nasal causes of snoring that are commonly encountered in an ear, nose, and throat practice:

Infection: Acute or chronic infections frequently cause nasal obstructions. Viral upper respiratory tract infections like the common cold are usually self-limiting and end in a couple of days, so that snoring may be temporary. Bacterial infections of the nose and sinuses, however, may cause persistent congestion and pressure in the head and face and are usually accompanied by increased nasal secretions and postnasal drip.

Allergy: About one person in ten suffers from allergic reactions during his life. Seasonal allergies, such as hay fever, are caused by sensitivity to grass, tree, flower, and weed pollens that drift through the air at certain seasons of the year. Perennial allergies, to house dust or cat hair and the like, usually produce persistent nasal congestion accompanied by copious watery secretions and bouts of sneezing.

Most upper respiratory tract allergies result in swollen mucous membranes inside the nose and, consequently, obstructed nasal breathing; hence snoring.

Drugs and medicines: Aspirin, oral contraceptives, and estrogens—to name but a few drugs—can bring about endocrine changes that affect the nasal air passages. Tobacco, as we now know, irritates the mucous membranes and impairs the protective action of the nasal hairs, called cilia. Decongestants (drops or sprays) can clear up the nasal airway, but relief is usually temporary. Repeated use actually irritates the membranes and creates further nasal obstruction. With each application the user benefits less from the decongestant, and that leads to increased dosage or frequency of use, or both. As a result, the user can become a "nose-drop addict" with increased nasal inflammation.

A number of drugs used in the treatment of high

blood pressure can also lead to chronic congestion and obstruction.

Irritants: Continuous exposure to such occupational irritants as dust or fumes or to environmental pollution can create inflammation of the mucous membranes in the nasal airway and thus, nasal obstruction. While we are beginning to realize the severity of the irritants around us,

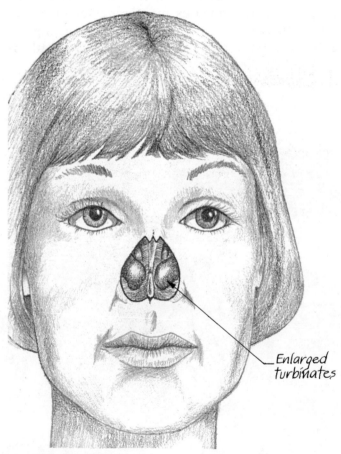

Enlarged turbinates

Environmental factors, allergies, and emotional upsets all can contribute to enlarged turbinates—and to snoring.

correcting the damage we've done and are doing to our air is an issue that will always demand monitoring and control.

Vasomotor rhinitis: This condition, which frequently brings patients into my office, is blamed on an imbalance in the autonomic (automatic) nervous system that controls the blood flow through the mucous membranes of the nose. In other words, the fine balance in the neural control of the mucous membrane somehow becomes disturbed through such factors as position, humidity, temperature, exercise, or emotion. The result is

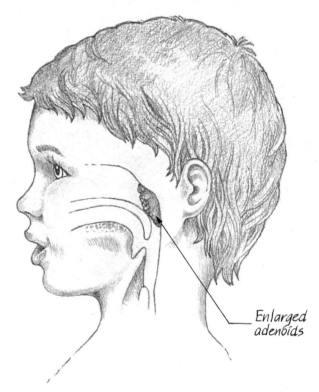

Enlarged adenoids

Snoring may be an early symptom of obstructive adenoids in the breathing passages.

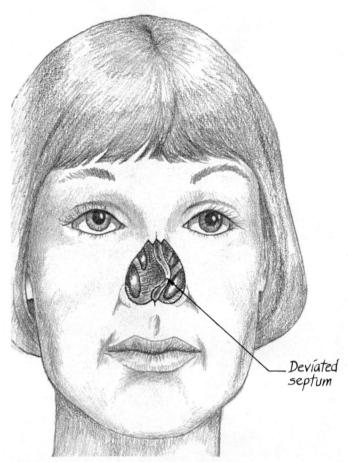

Deviated
septum

Deviated septum causing nasal obstruction.

swelling in the bony structures of the inside walls of the nose, called turbinates. The symptoms of vasomotor rhinitis are similar to those of certain allergies, where there is either persistent congestion or excessive drainage. The exact cause of vasomotor rhinitis is unclear, though the condition is often seen in people suffering from depression, chronic emotional stress, or anxiety.

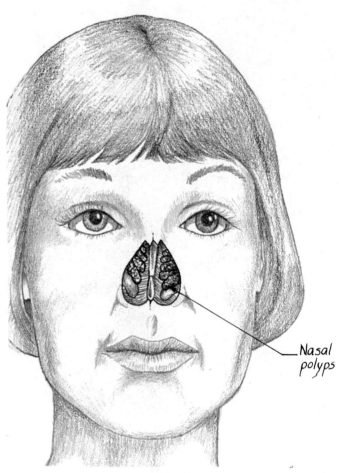

Nasal
polyps

Nasal polyps grow progressively larger, possibly leading to complete obstruction of airflow.

Growths and swellings: Obviously, tumors in the nose or sinuses, or enlarged adenoids can contribute to nasal congestion and obstruction, and one of the early symptoms may be increased snoring.

Anatomic deformities: Among the most common conditions in this group are a deviated nasal septum and nasal polyps, both of which can produce significant nasal obstruction.

The nasal septum is a bony and cartilaginous partition separating the two sides of the nasal cavity. Injury to the septum or asymmetrical growth during childhood can cause buckling of these structures, resulting in nasal obstruction.

Nasal polyps are localized swellings arising from the mucous membranes of the nose and sinuses. These pale, grapelike swellings tend to produce progressive nasal obstruction as they continue to grow inside the nose. The obstruction can range from partial to complete, and frequently there is secondary infection in the sinuses resulting in symptoms of chronic headaches and postnasal drainage. Physicians suspect that most polyps have an allergic basis.

Nasopharyngeal lesions: A variety of obstructive tumors can arise from the area behind the nose called the nasopharynx. These lesions usually cause progressive nasal obstruction. Other symptoms may include bleeding, pain, postnasal drainage, and, of course, snoring.

Why Do Men Snore More?

Throughout the investigation into the causes of snoring, one constant is that snoring occurs far more commonly in men than in women. Although the numbers vary according to the research, snoring is approximately ten times more common in men. But why?

We suspect that men have a greater tendency to build up bulky tissues which become filled with fat, get softer and more relaxed as they age, and therefore, contribute to snoring. This male characteristic is largely due to the action of a male hormone (androgen) that encourages increased appetite, weight gain, and salt retention—all of which can aggravate snoring. Physicians recognize the profile of a typical snorer as a large, heavily-built man in his forties or fifties who has gained weight and neglected regular exercise.

A female hormone (estrogen), on the other hand, is said to protect against the development of severe snoring in women by stimulating respiration. This is born out by the fact that the incidence of women snorers increases after menopause.

In summary, any factor that constricts or narrows the upper respiratory airway and brings the collapsible tissues into greater contact with the air flow is a cause of snoring—because snoring is the sound produced when these tissues begin to vibrate uncontrollably and rapidly as we breathe.

Recognizing the causes of snoring represents not only a breakthrough in the field of sleep medicine, but a valuable contribution to the well-being of snorers everywhere. Because when we understand causes, we can start to identify cures. And in that critical transition from causes to cures, snorers can be released from the frustrating world of gadgetry and bromides and brought into the scientific world of sound medical diagnosis and treatment.

Before we come to a discussion of that world, however, we must first understand the many side effects of snoring so we can decide *when* medical attention is required for the snorer and what sort it should be. Medical science has now come to realize that understanding and treating snoring can sometimes be more than merely treating a social annoyance—it can be saving a life.

CHAPTER 3

The Serious Side of Snoring

For some people, snoring can be much more than bad noise; it can be a sign of big trouble! Sometimes it is a symptom of an undetected medical condition. In other words, snoring often acts as nature's smoke alarm, alerting you to a health problem that may require medical attention.

Admittedly, not *all* the effects of snoring are serious. This amusing but pointed snore story appeared in the *New England Journal of Medicine:*

A 66-year-old man came to visit Neil Shear, M.D., of Toronto, complaining of pain and tenderness in his right calf. Finding no obvious cause for these symptoms, the doctor prescribed painkillers to help the patient through the next few days, telling him to come back if the pain became worse. "Several nights later," as Dr. Shear reported in his letter to the *Journal,* "the patient had just fallen asleep, when he was awakened by a sharp pain in the right calf, caused by a kick from his wife."

"Don't kick me there," he said. "That's just where my leg hurts."

"You were snoring again," she answered, "and that is where I always kick you to stop it."

The symptoms and ailments associated with snoring are often just as mysterious as this patient's calf pain. In fact, sleep disorders centers throughout the world demonstrate every day that snoring is not simply an isolated, irksome quirk but may be connected in some way to an underlying medical problem.

Tired from Snoring

In 1984, a medical clinic in Washington, D.C., studied the experiences of a group of severe adult snorers and their partners. As expected, these accounts included such complaints as "drives wife from bedroom" and "girlfriend won't marry him." But such comments as "falls asleep on the job," "naps while watching TV," "is drowsy all day," and "falls asleep eating dinner" were more intriguing from a medical viewpoint. These symptoms suggest that snoring is more than just a bothersome sound, but is somehow related to excessive tiredness.

It was hardly the first time sleepiness had been associated with some other medical condition. In 1837, *The Posthumous Papers of the Pickwick Club* by Charles Dickens told of a very fat boy who fell asleep and was "snoring feebly," while standing perfectly upright and knocking on a door. This character portrayal ultimately found its way into the medical literature. Nearly a century later, Sir William Osler, a renowned physician and professor of medicine at Johns Hopkins Medical School, coined the term *Pickwickian* for obese patients who exhibited excessive sleepiness.

But the correlation between sleepiness, obesity, and *snoring* was yet to be made.

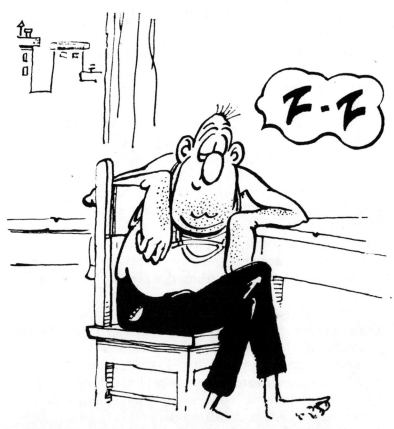

A night with obstructive sleep apnea leaves you groggy in the morning.

When Snoring Takes Your Breath Away

Finally, in 1965, the first report to make this connection appeared in the medical literature. It told of an obese patient who complained of constant tiredness and sleepiness during the day—and was a heavy snorer. His snoring was associated with periods when he would stop breathing. This led to the realization that some patients who had previously been diagnosed as having narcolepsy (a sudden, irresistible need to sleep) suffered instead from obstructed breathing, which resulted in episodes of asphyxiation during sleep, followed by excessive daytime sleepiness (EDS).

Based on this discovery, Elio Lugaresi, M.D., a renowned sleep researcher, proposed the phrase *hypersomnia with periodic apnea*—apnea meaning a cessation of breathing—for this condition in 1972. As an alternative description, he offered the more colorful *la maladie du gros ronfleur* (the illness of the heavy snorer). Then, in 1975, at an international congress on sleep-related disorders, sleep apnea and sleep apnea syndromes were finally chosen as the accepted medical terms for these conditions. Apnea is derived from the Greek, "for want of breath."

Snorers aren't the only people who experience periods of sleep apnea. Brief apneas of up to 10 seconds also occur during the sleep of healthy nonsnorers from infants to adults. Occurring fewer than 20 to 30 times during the night, these apneas are usually considered normal and are likely to increase with age or when alcohol or sedatives are consumed before going to bed.

With the development of sophisticated techniques to study sleep-related breathing disorders, researchers have been able to identify patterns of sleep apnea and classify them into several categories.

Obstructive sleep apnea (OSA): Breathing is blocked by closure or collapse of the tissues in the throat so that no air flows through the sleeper's nose or mouth despite his efforts to breathe.

Central sleep apnea: The movement of the diaphragm (the muscle separating the chest from the abdomen) is temporarily stopped. This type of apnea is usually associated with some abnormality within the central nervous system that controls breathing. One rare but tragic form of central sleep apnea is known as Ondine's Curse, caused by the primary failure of the automatic breathing center in the brain, sometimes resulting in sudden death during sleep. However, experts working in sleep clinics are convinced that many cases previously thought of as central sleep apnea are actually due to breathing obstruction. Over 90 percent of all sleep apneas are associated with upper airway obstruction; central respiratory failure without upper airway obstruction accounts for relatively few apneas.

Mixed sleep apnea: A condition present when obstructive and central sleep apnea coexist. From a practical point of view, mixed apnea is usually regarded as obstructive in nature.

There are some variations on this theme. We may see, for example, an incomplete form of apnea when the airflow is reduced by more than half. Known as hypopnea, this is regarded as having the same significance as apnea. Hypopneas are similarly classified as obstructive, central, or mixed.

Wake Up, Dear—
You're Choking!

Snoring and OSA do not develop hand in hand. Severe habitual snoring usually precedes the development of OSA. However, once the heavy snoring pattern is established, there is usually a progression in the severity of snoring as well as an increase in the number of times the snorer stops breathing during the night. With each of these repeated apneas, the sleeper becomes increasingly short of oxygen until each apnea wakes him. These are the moments that send the snorer's companion into a panic—the snorer appears to have stopped breathing! In fact, that's exactly what happens.

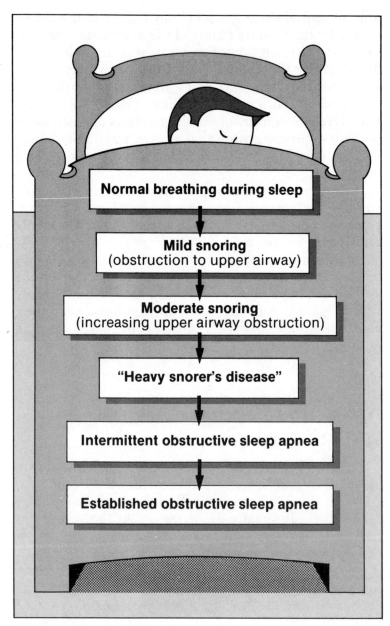

Development of obstructive sleep apnea.

When normal breathing resumes, the snorer overcomes the choking consequences of OSA and goes back to sleep, only to have the whole sequence repeat itself. In severe cases, these episodes can occur hundreds of times throughout the night.

In virtually all cases of OSA, the back of the throat (the pharynx) is the primary site of the obstruction. At some point, inhalation causes the soft tissues at the back of the throat to collapse enough to create airway obstruction. This area is narrowed during sleep by the combined effects of muscle relaxation, mucous membrane congestion, and the tongue being pulled backward by gravity.

Anatomical abnormalities in the upper airway, such as markedly enlarged tonsils or a very bulky tongue, can further the development of OSA, although most patients with this problem *do not* have these gross anatomical abnormalities in their upper airway. However, one or more of the conditions that cause snoring is usually present in patients with OSA and the majority of these patients are overweight.

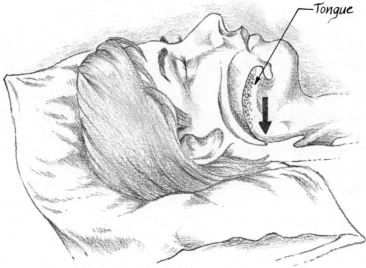

The tongue falls back during sleep.

We don't know exactly how obesity affects the upper airway but we do know that there is strong external pressure on the walls of the throat in those who have very thick necks. The floppy, easily collapsible pharynx in heavyset and heavy-snoring patients shows their snoring as an intermediate stage between a completely normal upper airway and the development of OSA.

Aging also produces flabbiness in the soft tissues of the upper airway, and coupled with the vibrations of snoring, these tissues eventually collapse enough to obstruct your airway.

Finally, any nasal obstruction can cause an additional vacuum effect in the back of your throat when you inhale, leading to collapse of your throat tissues. It's as if you were sucking the air out of a paper bag.

How Your Body Handles Apnea

When a snorer stops breathing during an episode of apnea, a number of chemical changes take place in his body. The oxygen level in his blood starts to drop (this is known as hypoxia), and the carbon dioxide level rises (hypercapnia) along with the degree of acidity in his blood. The effect on breathing is the same as if his head were being held under water.

The level of oxygen in the blood of a snorer experiencing OSA goes down as the duration of obstruction in his upper airway goes up. Of course, any chronic disease or thickening of the membranes in the snorer's lungs—such as seen in heavy smokers or asthmatics—compounds the oxygen shortage that occurs during each OSA event.

The rising level of carbon dioxide in the snorer's body during OSA episodes triggers that part of the brain controlling respiration to awaken the snorer and overcome the breathing obstruction. This wake period lasts a matter of seconds; hence the term *micro-arousal*. And the

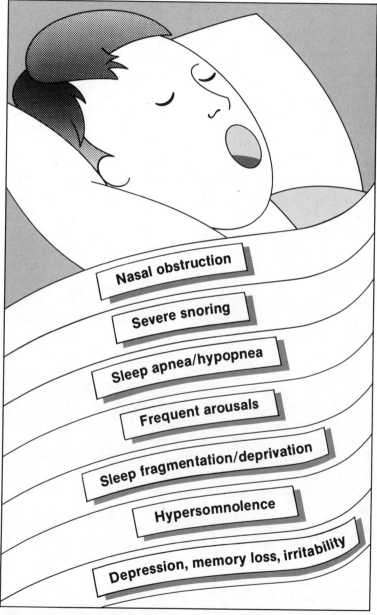

Consequences of nasal obstruction and sleep disturbance.

sleeper usually doesn't know that he has momentarily awakened. And even if he does know he is awake, he doesn't realize that it was due to a biological, lifesaving action. His anxious partner is often wide awake by now, nervously following the changing patterns—severe snoring . . . silence . . . breath holding . . . a deep gasp . . . restless body movements . . . falling back into a deep sleep—snoring resumes. And this cycle repeats itself throughout the night.

A snorer's sleep becomes fragmented by these recurring micro-arousals, which may occur hundreds of times during the night. Ironically, these awakenings get the snorer breathing again—and thus save his life—but seriously interfere with the quality of his sleep. Imagine how you would feel in the morning if your telephone rang throughout the night, waking you every 10 to 15 minutes. Researchers believe that sleep fragmentation/sleep deprivation and the interruption of the rapid eye movement (REM) phase of sleep accounts for many of the physical problems that characterize the sleep apnea syndromes.

Someone with a history of heart disease, for example, can further aggravate that problem if he snores heavily enough to cause OSA. The reduced oxygen and increased carbon dioxide that follow affect the sleeper's heart and blood vessels. Slowed heart rates and abnormal heart rhythms, as related to low oxygen levels as well as to acid-base changes in the blood, can sometimes lead to heart attacks and even cardiac arrest during sleep. If the snorer also suffers from narrowing of blood vessels to the heart (ischemic heart disease), the sleep apnea puts him at severe risk during the night.

Long-standing OSA that causes lowered blood oxygen levels and impairs functioning of the heart muscles may also cause cardiac failure.

When a large number of patients with established OSA were studied, over 70 percent demonstrated high blood pressure. This hypertension is probably due to a rise

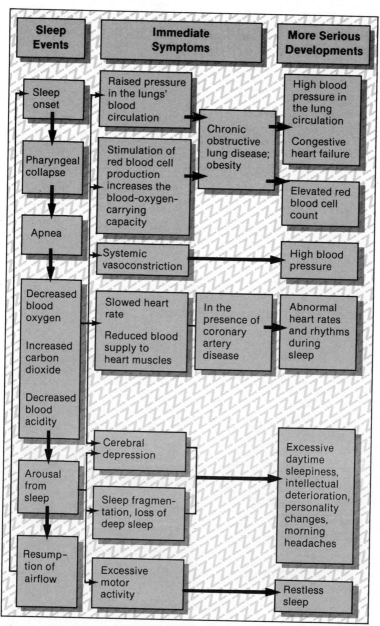

The causes and effects of obstructive sleep apnea.

in blood pressure during each obstructive apneic episode, which doesn't recede to normal levels during waking hours.

Diagnosis: Insomnia—Wrong!

The wake response during apnea episodes is associated with restlessness, often accompanied by excessive arm and leg movements. These fitful sleep interruptions, resulting from reduced levels of oxygen and REM sleep, contribute to many of the symptoms of OSA, including daytime sleepiness, mood changes, memory loss, and depression. Unfortunately, for the already suffering snorer, the symptoms that result from OSA are sometimes misdiagnosed as insomnia.

Morning headache is also a very common symptom among OSA sufferers. Doctors believe it is due either to high blood pressure or the dilating effects on the cerebral

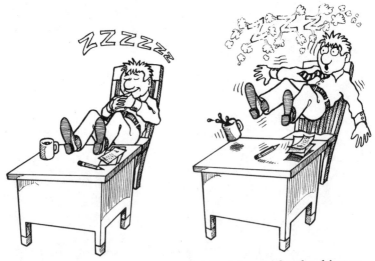

A good, loud snore keeps Gus awake all night—and wakes him up during his after-lunch snooze.

blood vessels that results from the abnormally high levels of carbon dioxide in the blood during the recurring apneas.

Impotence is another frequently misdiagnosed and stress-producing symptom of OSA. It occurs, we believe, from the combined effects of sleep deprivation and depression that come from a continued low oxygen state (hypoxia) similar to that seen in patients with chronic lung disease.

Approximately 80 percent of those with OSA admit to getting sleepy during the day. This is due to the hypoxia and sleep deprivation/fragmentation that escalate with the degree of obstruction at night, producing emotional symptoms such as mood changes, decreased intellectual function, and depression. Together with these mental and emotional changes, the physical incapacity produced by excessive daytime sleepiness (EDS) causes the snorer problems at work, invites automobile and occupational accidents, social difficulties, and can lead to problems in marriage and other relationships. One of my patients admitted driving 20 miles past his freeway exit because he had somehow put himself on automatic pilot. But perhaps the most remarkable example of hypersomnolence is the Las Vegas dealer who fell asleep, snoring uncontrollably, between poker hands, oblivious to the noise and excitement of the casino. Regrettably, these symptoms are frequently diagnosed as psychological rather than physiological in origin.

Sleep Apnea Results in Fuzzy Thinking

Problems in performing intellectual skills also plague long-time sufferers of OSA. For example, the *Wall Street Journal* reported the experience of Robert Legan, an indus-

Business Billed
for Sleep Disorders

Sleeping problems in the workplace—whether the result of irregular shifts or medical disorders—are costing companies an estimated $70 billion annually in lost productivity, huge medical bills, and avoidable industrial accidents. Sleep disorders, of course, are particularly frightening in areas affecting public safety. Researchers say that as more is learned about the economic toll of sleep disorders, companies will find they cannot afford to continue ignoring the problem. Megabucks are involved, and sometimes, lives.

The Wall Street Journal
(July 7, 1988)

trial physicist for Texas Instruments, who slept poorly over several years and, in the interim, lost the ability to solve abstract problems as well as he once could. "I'd be trying to construct an equation, and I'd have to go look in books," he said. "And even then, I'd have a hard time figuring out these things that I'd known two years before." Subsequent examination at a sleep disorders center revealed that Legan suffered from sleep apnea.

Unfortunately, we still don't know how often snoring leads to OSA. "We know that in this country," says David Fairbanks, M.D., of George Washington University School of Medicine, "about one person in eight snores. We don't know what percentage of snorers will eventually

Does Snoring Cut into Intelligence?

According to the results of an experiment conducted by A. Jay Block, M.D., snoring can interfere with your intelligence and your ability to think and act when awake.

Dr. Block's findings, which he discussed at a meeting of the American Society of Chest Physicians in Anaheim, California, in 1985, centered on heavy snorers recruited in an effort to determine the effect of oxygen deprivation on the brain. Each subject was hooked up to appropriate instruments during the night. The following morning the subjects were divided into three categories: those who never stopped breathing and never dropped their oxygen level; those who did so occasionally; and those who did so excessively.

IQ, memory, and verbal fluency all dropped in direct proportion to oxygen deprivation. In other words, those who stopped breathing most frequently during the night scored the lowest on tests given the following day for intelligence, reaction times, and visual coordination.

"I don't want to say that snoring makes you stupid," Dr. Block concluded, "but you may not be able to accomplish your whole potential. It may make you a little less smart."

It is significant that the majority of people tested were students or professors who were ordinarily required to function at a high intellectual level.

suffer from sleep apnea. We believe that apnea affects 2 to 3 million people across the country, and that every year 2 to 3,000 people die in their sleep because of it.''

During episodes of sleep apnea, the complete absence of airflow through the nose and mouth lasts for at least 10 to 15 seconds, and periods of 30 to 40 seconds are not unusual. In severe cases, they last as long as a 60 seconds, or even more. Apnea sufferers are alarmed, even horrified, to see these recordings on their sleep tests, and they frequently remark that they cannot hold their breath in the awake state for anywhere near the duration of their documented apneas.

The explanation is that the body's oxygen needs in sleep are lower than in the awake, active state. It's analogous to the low gasoline consumption of an idling automobile compared with the increased gas consumption of a car speeding down the freeway.

But many snorers don't experience apnea, and some nonsnorers may have OSA. A large group of patients with sleep apnea at Stanford University Sleep Disorders Clinic showed the following distribution of symptoms: 96 percent snored very loudly; 44 percent experienced excessive daytime sleepiness; 24 percent had depression; 36 percent demonstrated reduced intellectual function; 56 percent were hypertensive; 23 percent admitted to impotence; and 8 percent suffered from enuresis (bed-wetting).

Unfortunately, records show that apnea during sleep is more common among the general population than the experts once thought. In 1988, researchers at Uppsala University in Sweden mailed 4,064 questionnaires concerning sleep habits, snoring, and hypersomnolence to a random sampling of men aged 30 to 69 in one municipality. Of the 3,201 who responded, 690 admitted to habitual snoring; 236 experienced significant daytime sleepiness.

In the second phase of this study, 156 of these men were invited for overnight sleep testing, based on the severity of their symptoms. Sleep studies were eventually done in 61 respondents, confirming OSA in 15.

Applying these statistics to the general population, these researchers concluded that at the lower limits, OSA affects 1.3 percent of the men in Sweden between the ages of 30 and 69—over 25,000 people.

Another two-phase investigation into the prevalence of sleep apnea associated with hypersomnolence among industrial workers in Israel produced similar results. Although questionnaires were sent to workers of both sexes, all of the positive respondents were male. This study concluded that more than 3 percent of the male industrial workers were afflicted with sleep apnea.

When Lifestyle Leads to Snoring

Misdiagnosis of OSA in adults can have an equally profound effect on the health and psyche of the sufferer. Consider the case of Peter Jones, a 57-year old executive, who lived his life in the fast lane. His days were filled with corporate meetings and long-distance phone calls. Lunches were often three-martini, high-pressure affairs with corporate directors and executives of other companies.

Peter awoke with a dull headache every morning, but he had learned to live with it. Afternoons, however, were difficult for him. Returning to the office after lunch, he would nod off and have difficulty concentrating. Evenings were even worse. Peter had numerous social commitments—charity events, dinner parties, and activities at his country club—where alcohol flowed freely. He often caught himself drifting off to sleep during the after-dinner speeches.

Peter's hectic pace left him little time for exercise, other than an occasional Sunday golf game. And this was usually followed by drinks and dinner at the club.

When Peter returned home at night, he invariably fell into a deep sleep accompanied by severe snoring, an added source of marital stress in a relationship already strained by his frequent absences. Peter's wife had taken to sleeping in a spare room so she could get a good night's rest.

Peter's sedentary life began to show in weight gain. This caused even more snoring, worse morning headaches, and more daytime sleepiness.

Finally, realizing that both his health and his marriage were failing, Peter consulted an internist who diagnosed "overwork" and encouraged him to eat and drink more sensibly, put him on an exercise program, and prescribed a mild tranquilizer.

Though his weight dropped, Peter's symptoms worsened. His search for comfort eventually brought him to a lung specialist who had a special interest in sleep medicine. He recognized the symptoms of a sleep-related disorder in Peter and saw that tranquilizers were aggravating the condition by further relaxing his muscles and worsening an already severe case of OSA.

With expert treatment, Peter's suffering and accompanying despair were happily resolved.

Apnea in Children

Sleep disorders center studies show that snoring in children can also progress to OSA. In virtually every case, there is loud snoring punctuated by recurring periods of silence. After these periods of apnea, when no air flows through either the child's nose or mouth, you hear a broken, loud choking sound frequently accompanied by restless body movements. Parents describe these children as restless sleepers who tend to be difficult to arouse and who are disoriented and confused when awakened. These children may also wet the bed—usually due to a profound reduction in muscle tone (muscular hypotonia) as the child drifts into a deep level of sleep after numerous

Some Startling Statistics on Obstructive Sleep Apnea

● Approximately 3,000 people die in their sleep every year from causes directly related to obstructive sleep apnea (OSA).

● Two-thirds of people with sleep apnea have high blood pressure and one-third of people with high blood pressure have OSA.

● A tip for drowsy drivers: The second most common cause of driving fatalities, after alcohol, is excessive sleepiness. The risk is especially high for those who suffer from OSA—and this risk is heightened by the fact that this condition often goes undiscovered until after it causes a serious accident.

● Sleep-related disorders produce an estimated $70 billion loss to businesses each year from accidents, medical bills, and lost productivity.

awakenings. Unlike their adult counterparts, children who are severe snorers are usually not overweight. On the contrary, they tend to be thin and below their expected height and weight.

Changes in the intellectual ability of these children are common—attention lapses and inability to concentrate, for which they might be punished because their behavior is mistakenly regarded as daydreaming or indifference. Older children sometimes report morning headaches. Anatomical obstruction in the upper airway, frequently due to enlarged tonsils and adenoids, is among the most common causes of snoring and sleep apnea in children. Abnormalities in a child's facial skeleton, especially a small or recessed jaw bone, reduced muscle tone (as with Down's syndrome), and chronic nasal congestion (from allergy or infection) can also contribute to the development of sleep apnea.

Like adults, children with OSA have many symptoms that might be missed or misinterpreted by the attending physician. For example, poor weight gain and low energy levels are not unusual in children, nor are learning difficulties accompanied by a drop in school performance.

Johnny, the Snoring 5-Year-Old

Johnny White was a 5-year-old boy whose constant snoring had become the joke of the household—except to his older brother, who had to sleep in the same room.

Johnny looked like a child half his age. He was thin and spindly and had dark circles around his eyes. He always seemed tired and without energy, especially in the afternoons and evenings. Johnny became irritable and poked along at the table, pushing aside chunks of meat in favor of soft foods and liquids.

His parents had tried a number of remedies, including vitamin tonics and protein supplements, but to no avail. His pediatrician observed enlarged adenoids and referred Johnny to me. Johnny's adenoids were removed and on his first night home from the hospital he slept quietly for about 12 hours. Within a few weeks he gained some weight, had more energy during the day, no longer had the dark circles around his eyes, and regained his pleasant disposition.

Because snoring continues to be thought of as a nuisance rather than a medical problem, getting to the appropriate medical specialist is not always easy. The high blood pressure, impotence, depression, mood swings, and

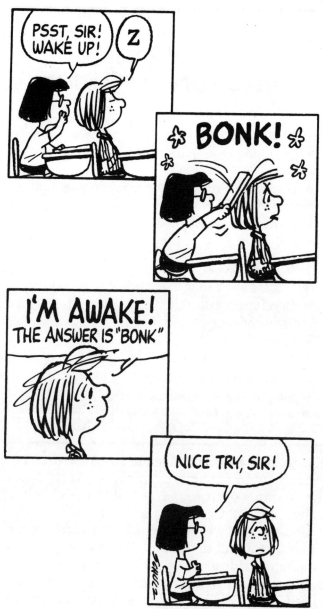

PEANUTS *Characters:* © 1966, 1971, *United Features Syndicate, Inc.*

Signs of Possible
Sleep Apnea in Children

While Asleep
- Loud snoring punctuated with recurring periods of silence.
- Disturbed sleep—restless movements, unusual body positions.
- Difficult to arouse.
- Bed-wetting.

While Awake
- Lethargic and slow to get going in the morning.
- Developmental delay, poor concentration, inattention, and moodiness.
- Excess daytime sleepiness.
- Morning headaches.
- Constant mouth breathing.
- Slow eating with poor appetite.
- Thin and underweight for age.

such are all too often misunderstood by the snorer or misdiagnosed by the physician, and years may be spent in futile attempts to fit square pegs into round holes. Now it's clear why OSA is called the darker side of snoring.

Understanding that snoring is a medical condition is the first step out of that cycle. The next step is to get the appropriate medical help. To do that effectively, the snorer needs a clear idea of how bad his snoring really is. He needs a quick but reliable test he can take on his own to determine his snoring level and whether or not there are any symptoms of associated sleep apnea.

CHAPTER 4

What's Your Snore Score?

Medical men who once dismissed snoring as little more than a hopeless nuisance now know better. Thanks to evidence provided by sleep researchers throughout the world, they are convinced that severe snoring is more than simply a social problem, but rather, a disease that can be treated. With this new attitude toward an old condition, we can start providing answers to questions that once were unanswerable.

- How severe is my snoring?
- How loud does it actually get during the night?
- What does it mean if: I choke and gasp between snores? My snores are punctuated by long periods of silence? I sleep fitfully, kicking out my arms and legs?
- When should I seek medical advice?
- When should I start to worry that my snoring might be causing sleep apnea (interrupted breathing between snores) or that the sleep apnea might be contributing to a health hazard?

I developed the following questionnaire to help you and your mate resolve these and other concerns you may have. I realize that it may be embarrassing to admit to loud snoring and even more difficult to admit to constant tiredness or depression. For most men it may be downright humiliating to discuss their own impotence. And many women are reluctant to come right out and say that their man snores outrageously. Such subjects do, after all, intrude into a most personal and private area—the bedroom. But it is important that you be completely frank in giving your answers.

I encourage you to think of the time you spend on this questionnaire as an opportunity to discuss a shared health concern with your mate. The purpose is to examine a medical condition with a view to obtaining help.

The Snore Score Questionnaire

Using the following scale, answer the questions by circling the number that most appropriately describes your situation: 1 . . . never; 2 . . . very infrequently; 3 . . . occasionally; 4 . . . often; 5 . . . always or almost always.

Snoring

1. How often have you been told you snore?   1 2 3 4 5

2. Does your snoring disturb your bedroom partner?   1 2 3 4 5

3. Does your snoring disturb others in the next room?   1 2 3 4 5

4. Has your snoring become progressively worse?   1 2 3 4 5

5. Do you snore when you sleep on your back?   1 2 3 4 5

6. Do you snore when you sleep in all positions?   1 2 3 4 5

7. Have you been told that you stop breathing for long periods between snores?   1 2 3 4 5

8. Has your snoring ever caused you to wake up suddenly?   1 2 3 4 5

9. Does your bedroom partner leave the room to sleep elsewhere because of your snoring?   1 2 3 4 5

10. Has your snoring caused you social embarrassment on vacations? At conferences? In motels?   1 2 3 4 5

Comments: If you scored 3 or more on questions 1 through 4, your snoring almost certainly interferes with your personal life.

With a score of 3 or more on questions 4, 7, and 8, there's a likelihood that you experience periods of apnea during your sleep. You should consult a physician.

If your answer to question 5 means you snore *only* when sleeping on your back, your snoring is probably due to the effect of gravity on the tissues of your upper airway rather than to any basic anatomical obstruction. You are what is called a positional snorer. Remedies that encourage you to sleep on your side or stomach may be sufficient.

If you scored 4 or more on question 6, your snoring is more than likely a result of some physical obstruction. You should see a physician for an examination of your upper airway.

A score of 3 or more on all questions in this section also indicates that apnea is very likely. You should see a physician and spend a night in a sleep disorders center so your snoring and sleep behavior can be observed and evaluated.

Sleep Habits

1. Does it take you a long time to fall
   asleep at night?   1 2 3 4 5
2. Do you wake up during the night?   1 2 3 4 5
3. Do you wake up before you've had a
   full night's sleep, unable to return to
   sleep?   1 2 3 4 5
4. Have you ever awakened choking or
   gasping for breath?   1 2 3 4 5
5. On awakening, do you still
   feel tired?   1 2 3 4 5
6. Is it difficult for you to awaken and
   get out of bed after sleeping?   1 2 3 4 5
7. Do you make frequent arm or leg
   movements during sleep?   1 2 3 4 5
8. Do you have bad dreams or
   nightmares?   1 2 3 4 5

Comments: Questions 4, 5, 6, and 7 deal with symptoms frequently associated with obstructive sleep apnea (OSA). If you score high on these questions *and* are a heavy snorer, I suggest you seek medical advice with a view to obtaining an overnight sleep test. The remaining questions in this section are inconclusive for sleep apnea and deal instead with sleep habits in general. However, if your answers are positive to most or all of the questions, you may have an underlying medical condition that adversely affects the quality of your sleep, and I suggest you seek appropriate medical attention.

Excessive Daytime Sleepiness

1. Do you feel tired during the day?   1 2 3 4 5
2. Do you take naps during the day?   1 2 3 4 5
3. Do you fall asleep watching TV, in church, or at the movies?   1 2 3 4 5
4. Have you ever fallen asleep while working (during a meeting or while operating machinery, for example)?   1 2 3 4 5
5. Do you experience drowsiness or a tendency to fall asleep while driving?   1 2 3 4 5
6. Have you ever been in a car accident because of drowsiness while you were at the wheel?   1 2 3 4 5
7. Are you experiencing any unexpected moodiness or increased irritability?   1 2 3 4 5
8. Are you aware of difficulty in concentrating or keeping your thoughts on track?   1 2 3 4 5

Comments: As with the preceding section, excessive daytime sleepiness (EDS) is not, in and of itself, an absolute indicator of severe snoring or sleep apnea. Anything that can cause a reduced oxygen level in the blood—such as fever and pain, heart failure, and any degree of emphysema, for example—can bring about EDS. One prominent cause of daytime sleepiness is narcolepsy. Those who suffer from this central nervous system disorder have a higher incidence of sleep apnea than occurs in the general population. Alcohol and other drugs can interfere with every level of sleep, resulting in sleep deprivation/fragmentation and EDS. Of course, psychological conditions, such as anxiety and depression, can also result in sleep loss and lead to EDS. The disorders of excessive sleepiness are numerous and are impossible to diagnose without a medical doctor's supervision. (See the box below.)

If your scores in the two previous sections indicate a strong likelihood of OSA, then high scores in this section (an average of 3 or more on each question) further support the suspicion of apnea. You should seek medical attention, since your sleep habits could be harmful to your health.

Disorders of Excessive Sleepiness

● Sleep apnea syndromes (obstructive, central, or mixed).

● Narcolepsy.

● Drug-related syndromes (excessive use of drugs or drug withdrawal).

● Nocturnal myoclonus (excessive muscle movement during sleep).

● Endocrine conditions such as hypothyroidism, diabetes, or hypoglycemia.

● Intermittent metabolic conditions such as premenstrual syndrome and pregnancy.

● Sleep drunkenness (prolonged and exaggerated transition from sleep to wakefulness).

● Congestive heart failure.

● Chronic lung disease.

● Psychological or behavioral causes (insomnia, jet lag, shift-work changes, depression, or anxiety).

Lifestyle

Answer the following questions Yes or No.

1. Are you a moderate to heavy smoker? Yes No

2. Do you eat large meals shortly before going to bed? Yes No

3. Do you have a nightcap (alcohol) before going to bed? Yes No

4. Is your snoring worse after those occasions when you've had several drinks? Yes No

5. Do you exercise regularly? Yes No

6. Do you take tranquilizers, sedatives, decongestants, or stimulants? Yes No

7. Do you drink large amounts of caffeinated beverages (coffee, tea, cola)? Yes No

8. Are you within your recommended body weight? Yes No

9. Has your snoring increased as a result of weight gain? Yes No

10. Does impotence disrupt your sex life? Yes No

Comments:

Question 1: Smoking is known to irritate the mucous membranes of the upper airway. It causes swelling and increased mucus production—both of which add to obstruction of the airway. This can cause snoring or make it worse.

Question 2: It requires a lot of energy to digest large meals, especially if they are rich in protein. Blood is diverted from your brain to your intestines to aid in digestion. This brings on a heavier sleep which results in increased muscle relaxation, vibration, and ultimate collapse of the pharyngeal tissues—all of which aggravates snoring. A distended stomach from overeating can interfere with movement of the diaphragm, which reduces respiratory movement and worsens apnea.

Questions 3 and 4: Alcohol is a potent central nervous system depressant, as it promotes muscle relaxation and upper airway collapse. It also depresses your arousal response to reduced oxygen levels. This can push a severe snorer into true OSA or aggravate the condition in one who already has it.

Question 5: Through exercise you increase and maintain muscle tone, which can overcome the tendency of the upper airway tissues to collapse.

Questions 6 and 7: Tranquilizers, sedatives, and decongestants are all central nervous system depressants, which have the same effect on snoring and apnea as alcohol does. Stimulants (such as caffeine) can interfere with the normal sleep cycle, often causing insomnia. When restful sleep finally comes, it tends to be deeper, accompanied by greater muscle relaxation, which encourages snoring.

Questions 8 and 9: There is a very strong correlation between snoring and gaining weight. Furthermore, virtually all sleep apnea sufferers are overweight. The mechanisms by which excess weight affects snoring and apnea are discussed in chapters 2 and 3.

Question 10: Research shows that a substantial number of patients with OSA suffer from a reduced sex drive and impotence. Scientists think it's due to the combined effects of the continued oxygen reduction, fatigue, and depression caused by sleep deprivation/fragmentation and the repeated apneas.

By now, you and your partner should have a better understanding of the snoring that disturbs your nights. In previous chapters we looked at the anatomical, physiological, and behavioral factors that contribute to the condition of snoring. We also acknowledged that loud and constant snoring is not simply a social nuisance, but, in fact, a medical condition that may pose a real threat to your health.

Admittedly, the snore score questionnaire results cannot provide a complete answer to all your concerns. But the quiz patterns should make you more familiar with your sleep habits and their possible medical implications. It should help prepare you to consult with a physician and to understand what issues he or she will examine, as well as how they will be considered.

The next step is to obtain medical advice. That can often be a daunting task, so let us discuss how to enter the medical system in search of answers, and where to begin.

CHAPTER 5

Selecting a Physician

If you snore severely or are the partner of someone who does, and you feel that some kind of help is needed to cut the constant noise, you can choose from a number of medical specialists trained for the job. During the past decade, a new specialty, sleep medicine, has arisen. It is practiced by physicians who take an interest in the medical problems that affect the body when it switches over to "automatic pilot" during sleep. These physicians are usually drawn from the fields of pulmonology, neurology, otolaryngology—and sometimes psychiatry—and they frequently work together as a team for the benefit of the patient with a sleep-related breathing disorder.

Generally, people consult first with their family physician or internist when they have a medical problem. Too often, those doctors have been unaware of the latest developments in treating sleep-related disorders. Until recently, medical schools rarely dealt with this subject in any depth. As I look back over my own schooling, I cannot remember the word snoring ever being mentioned. No wonder I was so insensitive to the anguish of wives who complained bitterly about their husband's snoring. Like many of my colleagues, I blithely passed the matter off by telling these women that if they really loved their mate, they would learn to live with the problem. We've all come a long way since then!

The Winds of Change

Changes have also occurred in the medical schools' courses, with lectures and discussions on sleep apnea and other sleep-related problems now being included in classes on pulmonary medicine or as part of a neurology program. Articles on sleep-related disorders now appear with increasing regularity in medical journals and publications to inform nonspecialists of advances in this field. Popular magazines and newspapers such as *Reader's Digest, Time, People,* and the *Wall Street Journal* have all recently published articles on this topic.

A logical place to begin solving any serious snoring problem is with a physician who has a special interest in sleep-related breathing disorders. This may be a medical subspecialist in the field of pulmonary or neurological medicine, or an ear, nose, and throat specialist. Ask your family physician or internist for the names of appropriate physicians who can treat snorers. If he or she can't help you, the local medical society or hospital should have the information you seek. See the back of this book for a list of regional sleep disorders centers.

While all ear, nose, and throat physicians are familiar with upper airway problems, not all are familiar with the modern treatments available for snoring and obstructive sleep apnea (OSA). Some of these physicians, for example, specialize in children's ear disorders, while others specialize in facial and cosmetic surgery. You need to find out if the physician you are referred to is prepared to treat snoring and related problems.

That First Phone Call

Once you've selected the appropriate physician, don't attempt to conduct an extensive interview over the phone. Here is why doctors don't welcome such a discussion during your initial call.

Medical reasons: To give any medical advice, a physician must have a firm grasp of the patient's individual health history and specific clinical findings. This can't be acquired through a phone call.

Professional reasons: Few health questions have quick and easy answers; we want to speak at some length with the physician about our problem. But the patient who is in the office by appointment is understandably annoyed if his or her time is interrupted frequently by extended phone calls.

Legal reasons: The current climate of litigation makes physicians wary of providing detailed information over the phone to people they have never seen. For example, a lawyer might call on behalf of a hostile insurance company, but not identify herself as such. Or a patient may want to gain information that could be used against another physician.

What *can* you do? Call each physician on your resource list and ask the receptionist the following questions:

- Does Dr. _____ treat sleep-related breathing disorders and OSA?
- Does Dr. _____ conduct evaluations of snoring?
- Does Dr. _____ work in conjunction with a sleep disorders center?
- Is Dr. _____ familiar with the medical and nonsurgical treatments for snoring and OSA?

- Has Dr. _____ performed many surgeries for snoring?
- If Dr. _____ is a medical specialist, does he work in association with a surgeon trained in the modern surgical procedures for treatment of OSA?

If the answers to these questions indicate that the physician has an interest and involvement with snoring, then, using whatever other criteria are relevant for you—location, fees, availability—make an appointment for a consultation.

The Previsit Questionnaire

Before your first visit, or in the physician's office, you will receive a questionnaire regarding your general health and sleep history. It will usually include the following:

- Age, sex, weight, height, and recent weight gain.
- General health and surgical background (previous illnesses, surgeries, hospitalizations, and current medications).
- Personal history regarding diet, exercise, smoking, and alcohol.
- Ear, nose, and throat history (nasal problems, allergies, infections, and previous surgery on the tonsils, nose, or sinuses).
- Snoring history (loudness and pattern of the snoring, the amount of disturbance it produces [Does it awaken others? The snorer?], recent changes in intensity and pattern of snoring [Does the snorer stop breathing during the night?], body positions in which snoring occurs

[Are there excess body movements during sleep?], history of snoring in other individuals in the family, and frequency of snoring [Does it occur intermittently or throughout the night?]. Do the use of tranquilizers, other medications, or alcohol increase the snoring?)

● Sleep habits (estimated number of sleep hours, number of awakenings during the night, episodes of choking and gasping, difficulty getting up in the morning, and tiredness upon awakening).

● Excessive daytime sleepiness (sleepiness that causes constant fatigue, mood changes or depression, memory loss, personality change, accidents, or unusual sleep behaviors, such as falling asleep readily at church or the movies, or taking several daytime naps).

The Consultation— What to Expect

The initial visit is the appropriate time to ask your in-depth questions and to express your concerns. Now you are paying for a consultation. Consult!

Because the first step toward the diagnosis and treatment is made during this visit, I advise that the snorer's bedroom partner accompany him or her to the office. The companion can provide invaluable information for the doctor by describing the snoring in colorful terms that may not have been voiced before ("earthquake snoring," "baritone saxophone snoring," "big league snoring").

Your evaluation should include a complete physical—with special attention paid to your blood pressure, heart, and lungs—as well as a detailed examination of your upper respiratory tract. Usually these tests are not conducted by one physician; therefore you should not be surprised if you are referred to other specialists to complete your evaluation. Blood tests will also be performed and X-rays taken of your chest.

Of course, the study of the upper airway is an important part of this examination. Special attention will be paid to any abnormality or obstruction in the nasal airway, the area behind the nose (nasopharynx), the throat, larynx, and the region behind the tongue (hypopharynx).

Special instruments are required for this part of the examination, which is usually done by an ear, nose, and throat specialist. The physician uses a headlight or reflecting head-mirror, together with a nasal speculum to examine the inside of your nose for obstructions such as a deviated nasal septum, polyps, or enlarged nasal turbinates (the bones on the inside walls of the nose). Then the doctor will examine your mouth and oral cavity, taking special note of the size and position of your tongue, the presence of tonsils (their size and any intrusion they make on the airway), the length of the uvula, and the size and position of the folds of tissue in the soft palate on either side of the uvula.

The area in the back of the nose (nasopharynx) is examined with either a reflecting mirror or a fiber-optic nasopharyngoscope—a narrow, flexible tube that is inserted into your nose after preparing the mucous membranes with a local anesthetic and decongestant. It allows your physician to examine the nasal airway and the recesses in the back of your throat. Using this instrument, your doctor will usually be able to find any infection or obstructing lesion.

Searching the Sinuses

We know that nasal congestion or obstruction can cause or aggravate snoring. It also can contribute to the development of OSA. Additionally, chronic infection in

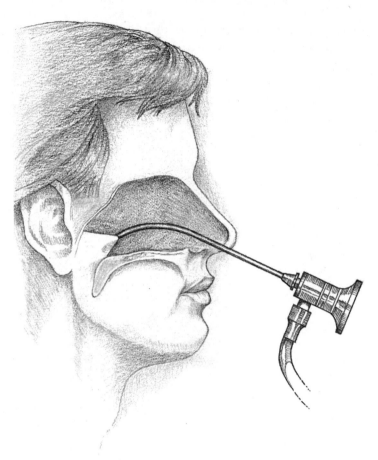

The fiber-optic endoscope allows for a detailed examination of the nose and nasopharynx.

the air-containing cavities in the bones of the face or skull (paranasal sinuses) can produce continuing symptoms of nasal congestion, increased nasal drainage, postnasal drip, and headache that together are sometimes referred to as "the cold that never goes away." More common in cooler climates, chronic sinus infection can affect people of all ages. Therefore, attention to the sinuses should be an integral part of the upper respiratory examination.

With the flexible endoscope, your physician looks for

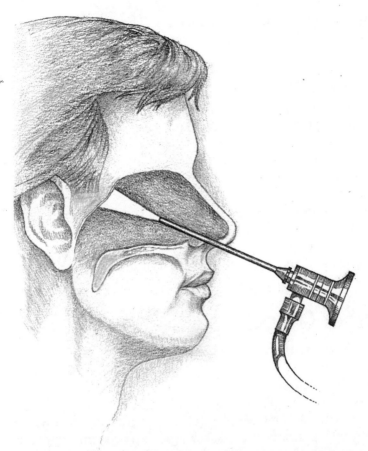

Examination of the nose with a rigid endoscope allows for a more detailed examination of the sinuses.

any nasal obstruction, such as a deviated septum or nasal polyp, which may contribute to chronic sinus disease. He or she also looks for increased secretions in the nose or nasopharynx, as this may be a sign of underlying sinus infection.

A more detailed examination of the sinuses may be done in your physician's office by spraying your nose with a decongestant and topical anesthetic solution and using a *rigid* endoscope to visualize the areas from which the sinuses drain into the nasal cavity. The optical clarity of this instrument allows the doctor to detect even relatively minor changes in the nose and sinus cavities; changes that may indicate underlying infection.

To complete the nasal examination, your doctor may order a special X-ray of the sinuses called Computerized Tomography (CT scan). In many cases, conventional X-rays may not show any evidence of sinus disease, whereas the CT scan provides finely detailed images of each sinus, from the frontal sinus in the forehead back to those at the base of the skull.

A radiologist usually interprets the CT scan images, working in collaboration with your physician. Once an abnormality is identified by the CT, your doctor will discuss and recommend the appropriate medical or surgical treatment for you.

Other Checkpoints

Physicians have come to understand the close association between OSA and chronic lung disease. Many snorers are heavyset, overweight individuals and are also heavy smokers. Their impaired lung function only worsens a mild case of OSA. Therefore, lung studies, known as pulmonary function tests, are especially recommended if you smoke and your Snore Score indicates the likelihood of OSA. Your doctor will test you when you are standing and lying down, in an attempt to reproduce the positions in which OSA occurs.

Your examination should also include an accurate assessment of the cardiovascular system. It's customary to record your resting blood pressure, taken while standing and supine, as well as to order an electrocardiogram (EKG). Your examining physician may also recommend an effort EKG, known as a treadmill test.

Although not routine, measurements may also be made between fixed bony points on the skull, taken from your X-rays. This test, called cephalometry, is now being given in a number of university hospitals and sleep research facilities. Cephalometry attempts to correlate the relationship of the anatomical structures in a person's head and neck with the site and level of the upper airway obstruction. These measurements help to determine sources of existing obstruction and to predict the tendency to develop airway obstruction during sleep, as well as aiding the physician in selecting appropriate medical or surgical procedures.

Your initial examination may provide your physician with the information needed to determine an effective medical treatment for your snoring. However, if you do need further investigation of your sleep habits, the doctor will usually prescribe an overnight sleep study. You will be pleased to learn that although the equipment used in a sleep disorders center is quite complex, the evaluation process is quite painless.

In fact, you will be able to sleep right through it!

CHAPTER 6

The Sleep Disorders Center:

A Test to Sleep Through

Two decades ago, only a few medical researchers were interested in sleep-related disorders, and specialized facilities for patients suffering from these problems were scarce. This situation changed dramatically in the early 1970s as more people sought help for disorders associated with sleep. In 1987, the American Sleep Disorders Association was established to set standards and provide certification and guidance for the rapidly emerging sleep disorders centers and their staffs.

Today, people with severe snoring problems can go to any of a number of knowledgeable physicians and sophisticated sleep disorders centers in all parts of the country, and, in fact, throughout the world. These facilities follow established standards as do the three basic groups of professionals involved: physicians associated with sleep disorders clinics, scientists doing basic sleep research, and technicians skilled in the administration of sleep testing.

If you or your partner snore and an overnight sleep study is recommended, you will no doubt have a number of preliminary questions about sleep disorders centers in general and your own study in particular. I will take you through a night in a so-called sleep lab so you can see exactly how such a study is conducted. But first, let's discuss some of the preliminary concerns you may have.

Here are some of the questions patients most often ask. They will, I believe, include most of your own.

- What is a sleep disorders center?
- Should I have a sleep test before seeing a physician?
- When is a sleep study recommended for a snorer?
- When is a sleep study not recommended for a snorer?
- Must a sleep disorders center be accredited?
- What are the costs, and which of them will my medical insurance cover?

Let's consider each of these questions more closely.

What is a sleep disorders center?

Housed within a hospital or medical center, a sleep laboratory—or sleep disorders center—is a diagnostic and short-term outpatient treatment facility established to study some or all of the following:

1. Difficulties in falling asleep.

2. Difficulties in staying asleep, due, for example, to sleep-related breathing disorders.

3. Abnormal behaviors during sleep (called parasomnias), such as sleepwalking, nightmares, and night-terrors.

4. Medical disorders associated with sleep, not occurring during waking hours, including abnormal movements during sleep, such as the restless legs syndrome.

5. The success and effectiveness of various medical and surgical treatments for one or more of the above disorders.

As a facility in a hospital or medical center, a sleep disorders center is supervised by a staff of specialists drawn from such disciplines as pulmonary medicine, neurology, psychiatry, and psychology. In addition, the center's supervisory staff includes an accredited polysomnographer (sleep study specialist) whose responsibility is to train technologists, oversee data gathering, supervise the various tests, and provide reports on the patients who are studied. The sleep lab is staffed by technologists who are specially trained in gathering reliable sleep data. Consultants—specialists in ear, nose, and throat problems (otolaryngologists), internal medicine, and cardiology—often complement this team.

Should I have a sleep test before seeing a physician?

No. You won't be permitted to do so. Because a sleep disorders center is part of a medical facility, an overnight sleep study is considered a medical evaluation and requires a physician's referral.

When is a sleep study recommended for a snorer?

A physician will recommend an overnight sleep study when:

1. You snore loud enough to disrupt the well-being of your bedroom partner on a consistent basis.

2. Your initial medical and sleep history evaluation reveals indications of suspected sleep apnea.

3. You suffer from excessive tiredness or sleepiness during waking hours.

Most people seek medical help for their snoring because it *has* become disruptive. That's why an overnight stay at a sleep disorders center is commonly recommended for most patients with severe snoring or other sleep disorders as a follow-up to preliminary findings.

When is a sleep study not recommended for a snorer?

If you are an occasional or mild snorer, without any of the symptoms commonly associated with obstructive sleep apnea (OSA), you may be advised to lose weight, exercise, or reduce any medications you are taking before having an overnight study. If your snoring has not diminished after three months or so, you will then probably be advised to have this test.

Must a sleep disorders center be accredited?

Accreditation of a sleep disorders center refers to the broad range of diagnostic capacities that a facility can offer. It identifies such a center as having the capability to study a full spectrum of sleep disorders, such as narcolepsy, nighttime seizures, insomnia, nightmares, bedwetting, sleepwalking, and impotence, as well as ensuring high medical standards.

Unlike studying some of these more complex disorders, monitoring snoring and testing for sleep apnea are fairly straightforward procedures. Any established sleep disorders center—accredited or nonaccredited—should be able to do it. What *is* important is that the testing be carefully done by trained personnel and that the results represent a true and accurate evaluation of the problem.

However, sleep disorders center accreditation may be an important financial factor. Before being admitted to any sleep disorders center, check with your insurance carrier to see if your policy will cover the overnight study. Most do, but ask if the facility must be accredited for coverage.

What are the costs, and which of them will my medical insurance cover?

Your medical insurance will probably cover the cost of the following:

- The initial office evaluation, including history and physical examination.
- Additional office tests, such as X-ray, electrocardiogram (EKG), and blood tests.
- Overnight sleep study tests.

Medical costs vary from county to county and from state to state, but the following represents the broad range of current charges:

- Complete polysomnography (all-night sleep evaluation): $700 to $1200.
- Ambulatory sleep monitoring test: $400 to $700

Some insurance companies hesitate to cover testing for snoring alone, but will usually do so on the strength of a physician's opinion that the snoring might be a symptom of a sleep-related breathing disorder.

I hope this answers some of your concerns. When questions are asked, everybody benefits. Becoming actively involved in your medical care is invaluable for you and the treating physician. We must ask questions at every step along the way so we can develop complete trust in each other. This book attempts to provide the information you need in order to ask the right questions.

An Overnight Sleep Study

Your doctor has reviewed your sleep history and clinical findings with you and has recommended an overnight sleep study. What should you expect while you're there?

An overnight sleep test is unlike most other medical evaluations. For one thing, you can sleep right through it! Also, there are no injections, anesthetics, or incisions, and there is no pain or discomfort. All you need to do is sleep in your natural way.

When the appointment with the sleep disorders center is made, you will be asked to come in a few hours before your usual bedtime. Ordinarily, you will have received a questionnaire and instructions concerning what you should bring with you (pajamas, toothbrush, robe, customary medications, and usual reading material).

You will see that the sleep center's questionnaire contains many of the questions that were included in your physician's preliminary evaluation. This redundancy is not due to a lack of communication between your physician and the center, it's just that the sleep center wants to have your medical information on its standard forms.

At the center, a member of the staff, usually the nighttime technologist, will greet you and take you to your room—a cross between a hotel room and a hospital room. There the technologist will explain the nature of the test, tell you what to expect, show you what will be done, and demonstrate the equipment to be used. Then he or she will attach the monitoring devices to your body.

You will learn that the *polysomnogram* (all-night sleep evaluation data) is recorded on a polysomnograph and will be interpreted by a physician, usually a certified clinical polysomnographer. The sophisticated equipment used on you will monitor your brain waves, heart rhythms, respiration, muscle tone, blood oxygen levels, and body movement throughout the night.

After you change into your nightclothes, the technologist attaches the monitoring equipment to your face, head, and body, using a special paste to ensure a firm seal for the electrodes. The wires from these monitoring sensors are plugged into a wall-jack in your room, and the information they carry is transmitted through a central line to a polysomnograph machine in an adjacent room— where your sleep study can be observed unobtrusively by the technologist.

This monitoring equipment may cause anxiety in some people. To dispel any apprehensions it might provoke, let's take a closer look at the various sensors and explain their purpose:

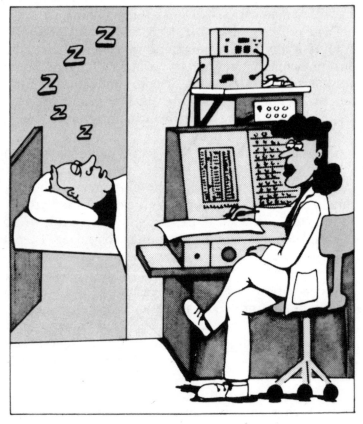

Monitoring equipment transmits data to an adjacent room, where it is recorded for evaluation by a medical specialist.

1. Electrodes are attached to your scalp to monitor brain waves. That's why you were asked to shampoo your hair before coming to the sleep lab; an oily residue might prevent good contact between the electrodes and the scalp. Don't worry. Your hair won't be shaved; the electrodes are merely glued onto your head in positions that correspond to points on the underlying cerebral cortex. This recording of brain wave activity is called an electroencephalogram. It records the phases of sleep and their association with snoring and apnea.

2. Leads are attached to your chest to measure your heartbeats for both rate and rhythm. These recordings, called electrocardiograms, are to detect any irregularity of heart rate or rhythm (called tachyarrhythmia) that might be associated with sleep apnea.

3. Electrodes are placed on your chin to record muscle tone. These recordings are known as electromyography (EMG) and are intended to measure the changes in muscle tension and muscle tone that occur during the different phases of sleep.

4. Electrodes are placed at the corners of your eyes to measure eye movement. These recordings, called electrooculography (EOG), correlate your snoring with different phases of sleep—rapid eye movement (REM) sleep and non-rapid eye movement (NREM) sleep, which we discussed in chapter 2.

5. Temperature-sensitive devices are taped under your nostrils and mouth to record your breathing rate and the volume of the inhaled air. Called thermistors, these sensors detect any change in air movement. They are sensitive enough to record shallow breathing or cessation of inspiration.

6. Electrodes are applied to each leg to monitor muscle activity. They record the presence of excessive leg movement during sleep, frequently observed in patients suffering from sleep apnea.

7. Bands are secured around your chest and abdomen to record thoracic and abdominal expansion and contraction as you breathe. Called strain gauges, these bands stretch and measure the amplitude of each breath, allowing the technologist to distinguish between normal quiet breathing, heavy snoring, and the different types and degrees of apnea and hypopnea.

8. To record blood oxygen saturation, a clip known as a transcutaneous pulse oximeter is attached to your earlobe or finger. This device records, through your skin, the percentage of oxygen saturation in your arterial blood and indicates any decrease in saturation associated with breathing interruptions.

These various devices continuously record your physical and physiological patterns during your overnight sleep study. Though they may differ in number, appear-

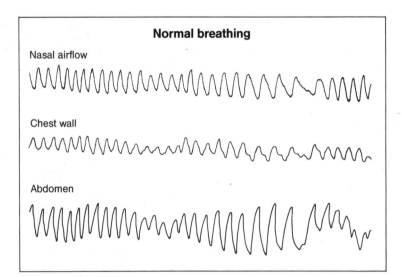

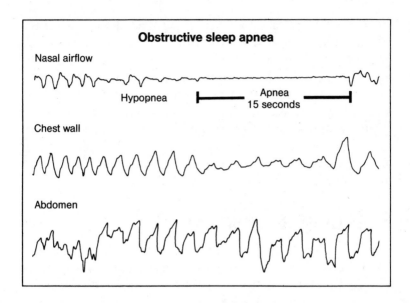

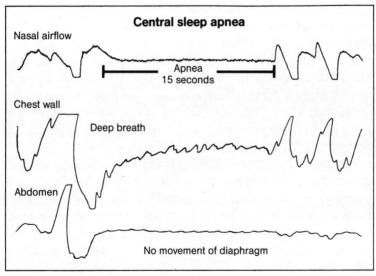

Recorded respiratory patterns during sleep.

ance, and body placement from one sleep disorders center to another, they will be functionally identical, monitoring the fundamental sleep behavior that needs to be studied in an effort to bring your disruptive nights to an end.

Although the monitoring equipment is somewhat confining, you will be able to turn over in bed and assume your natural sleeping positions. You will be asked to use the bathroom before the sensors are attached, but if you have to answer nature's call during the actual test, the technologist will provide a bedpan.

Listening to Learn More

In addition to the sensors I have described, you will notice that there is a microphone in the room. This allows the technician to listen to your breathing and assess and record the degree of your snoring. It also allows you to communicate with the technician, should you need anything during the night.

There will probably be a TV/video camera and a one-way mirror in your room for further observation. The camera is usually placed on the opposite side of the bed from the mirror. It enables the technician to observe your behavior continually and confirm that the sensors remain attached, should you turn over in your sleep.

Some sleep disorders centers—not all—make an audiotape of your snoring, or an audiovisual tape of the complete sleep sample. Because snoring is the primary symptom of nocturnal upper airway obstruction, it is important that the intensity of your snoring (loudness, frequency, and duration) be accurately studied. The result is better patient evaluation, improved treatment planning, and more accurate assessment of the success of treatment methods. It also provides objective documentation for your physician.

The technique for measuring and recording the sounds of snoring and airway obstruction is known as sleep sonography. Typically, a microphone is placed near the snorer's head and the electrical signal is fed into a noise analyzer and tape recorder. The analyzer classifies signals from the microphone, transferring this data to a computer for display and storage, in both graphic and tabular form.

When you are ready to go to sleep, the technologist on duty turns off the lights (remember, you can't leave the bed) and watches the brain waves recorded on the polysomnograph, noting the exact time sleep occurs. Throughout the rest of the night, the sensors send signals to the polysomnograph, and these signals are converted into electrical impulses, appearing as wavy lines on the continuous sheets of paper fed into the machine. During a single night's sleep recording, more than one-half mile of paper may be covered with squiggles and waves.

In the morning, you will be asked questions about how you slept, including estimates of how long it took you to fall asleep, how often you awakened, and how this night compared with a normal night's rest at home. The purpose of the questions is to correlate the electronically recorded information with your own impression of the experience.

The lab technologist helps you remove any electrode paste from your scalp and body. Then, after a shower and a welcome cup of coffee, you will be on your way, early enough to be on time for work.

At the conclusion of your sleep study, the data from the polysomnograph is processed by a computer, calculating the time it took you to fall asleep, the time in each sleep stage, awakenings, breathing patterns, apneic episodes, changes in heart rate, and final awakening. This report, customarily generated by a medical specialist associated with the sleep laboratory, is sent to your referring physician several days or weeks after the sleep study. Before going on to review a typical sleep test report with you, I should mention that in rare instances a sleep study may have to be repeated for the following reasons:

1. You were unable to sleep at all.

2. You and your physician feel that the test is not a truly representative sleep sample. (You slept poorly, had nightmares, touches of insomnia, or a fitful sleep.)

3. You slept quietly through the night and never snored, despite a history of severe snoring that led to the test in the first place.

4. There were technical problems (for example, a dislodged sensor went unnoticed) that prevented achieving a complete and accurate test recording.

A Sleep Study Report

To illustrate a typical sleep disorders center evaluation, I'll review the case report of a patient I'll call Bill. He consulted with me because he had a history of severe nighttime snoring in all body positions. His wife became concerned with his irregular breathing, his choking sounds, and his restless sleep behavior. He admitted to some daytime drowsiness, occasionally dozing off in church or at the movies. A physical examination showed that Bill was in good health, although slightly overweight. An examination of Bill's nose and throat revealed no abnormality other than slight enlargement of his tonsils. Because of his obviously disruptive sleep behavior, I recommended that Bill undergo a sleep study, and the following report came to me from the sleep center:

> This 48-year-old male was referred because of complaints of excessive snoring throughout the night, irregular breathing during sleep, and episodes

A Fully Operational
Sleep Disorders Center

An accredited facility will provide the following:

1. Two or more separate sleeping rooms, equipped with two-way intercoms.

2. Each room equipped with polysomnograph machines to record the specific functions being monitored on 8 to 14 channels.

3. An accurate method for all-night monitoring of arterial blood oxygen, such as a transcutaneous ear oximeter (a device attached to your ear which measures blood-oxygen ratios through the skin).

4. One full-time technician who conducts polysomnography (sleep recording) during the night.

5. One full-time daytime technician who prepares for the nightly studies, scores records, and conducts daytime testing.

6. An office to process and store laboratory data.

7. A clinical coordinator to facilitate patient referrals for associated studies such as pulmonary function, cardiac studies, and electroencephalograms.

8. An accredited clinical polysomnographer (a medically qualified sleep evaluator who may be an M.D. or a Ph.D.).

9. A full-time physician with expertise in sleep physiology to assure continuity of medical care in the evaluation of sleep disorders patients.

10. Good working relations with associated clinical services of cardiology, neurology, otolaryngology, pediatrics, psychiatry, pulmonary medicine, and urology.

11. In-hospital emergency code coverage whenever sleep patients are monitored.

of suspected apnea associated with body move-
ments. He apparently suffers from a degree of
daytime drowsiness.

An overnight sleep study was performed in our
sleep center, and the patient was studied in the
usual manner with bipolar electroencephalograph
leads. Nasal and oral thermistors and thoracic and
abdominal strain gauges were applied. An earlobe
oximeter was attached. The study is of good techni-
cal quality and easily interpreted. The patient had
adequate amounts of REM sleep for interpretation.

The patient commenced sleeping without dif-
ficulty and was observed to snore throughout the
entire sleep sample. He slept on his back for most of
the study, turning occasionally onto the left side.
Total sleep time was 362 minutes. During this
sample, 180 respiratory disturbances (apneic epi-
sodes) were observed and recorded. These episodes
varied in duration from 15 to 41 seconds, with an
average length of 26 seconds. During these apneas,
the pulse rate dropped to below 50 beats per minute,
and the blood oxygen saturation levels fell as low as
68 percent saturation.

Comment: *This patient is a severe snorer who*
has significant obstructive sleep apnea (OSA). The
apneas are associated with marked reduction in
blood oxygen saturation levels as well as bradycar-
dic episodes (slowing of the heart rate).

To understand the significance of this report we need
to familiarize ourselves with the classification of OSA
shown in the accompanying table.

The Apnea Index (also known as the Respiratory Disturbance Index) referred to in this table represents the
average number of times a patient stops breathing for
more than 10 seconds in each hour of sleep during the
test. Bill slept for 6 hours and had 180 apneas, resulting in
an Apnea Index of 30 (180 divided by 6 = 30).

Measuring the Severity of Obstructive Sleep Apnea (OSA)

OSA	Snoring	Daytime Sleepiness	Apnea Index	Blood Oxygen Desaturation (percent)	Heart Rate and Rhythm Changes
Simple	Yes	No	6–10	85 or more	No
Mild	Yes	No	11–30	75–84	No
Moderate	Yes	Occasionally	30+	50–74	No
Severe	Yes	Yes	30+	below 50	Yes

Here's how I interpreted the sleep lab report to Bill: "Based on your constant loud snoring, the presence of your daytime sleepiness, the number of apneic episodes recorded in your study, your oxygen desaturation levels, and the changes in your heart rate during sleep, I would say that you are a severe snorer who is suffering from a moderate degree of obstructive sleep apnea."

What Bill's sleep history, his daytime behavior, and his wife's observations had suggested, the sleep center's data had now confirmed. We were now able to consider appropriate corrective measures.

Ambulatory Home Monitoring

Now I want to discuss a more informal but nonetheless accurate sleep evaluation procedure that plays an increasingly prominent role in the diagnosis and treatment of sleep-related breathing disorders. This test is conveniently administered at home in the privacy of your bedroom.

While sleep disorders centers are rapidly multiplying (some authorities estimate that in the United States alone they number around 5,000), they aren't yet available in all parts of the country and might never be. But not everyone who snores needs to go to one. Several years ago, portable monitoring devices were developed, enabling a patient to obtain nighttime sleep study data at home. Known as an ambulatory monitoring system, it is a microcomputer designed for continuous analysis of information from as many as ten physiological sensors. This small, lightweight system is fitted and adjusted at your home by a technician who returns to collect the equipment at the end of the study. The data are collated and a report is generated for your physician.

Worn on a belt or placed next to the bed, this ambulatory monitoring system records the following data:

1. Heart rate changes and arrhythmias.
2. Blood oxygen saturation levels.
3. Nasal air flow.
4. Thoracic and abdominal expansion (respiratory efforts).
5. Body movements.

Recent advances in this technology allow for recording EOG (for eye movement), EEG (for REM and non-REM sleep differentiation), and EMG (for recording muscle tone).

Although these home-use devices cannot substitute for all the comprehensive testing you can get in a sleep lab, sleep researchers acknowledge that ambulatory monitoring plays an increasingly valuable role in the study of sleep-related breathing disorders. When the physician suspects a mild to moderate degree of apnea, and by medical history can exclude other sleep-related disorders, the ambulatory monitoring system may be a useful and less expensive way to document and measure the apnea. Some patients feel that because this test is done right in their bedroom, it represents a more natural and accurate sample of their sleep habits.

Because the home monitoring study is essentially a simpler test and requires less equipment and fewer personnel, it is less expensive than a sleep laboratory, and this is certainly a consideration. Many insurance companies provide coverage for these home-based tests, but you should determine this before having the study.

At present, the following concerns exist regarding the use of ambulatory monitoring systems:

● The study is less complete than that produced by a traditional sleep disorders center stay.

● The absence of a technical observer during the test may detract from its accuracy—for example, a sensor may become dislodged during sleep.

● Medically trained personnel are not at hand in the event of an emergency such as cardiac arrest during sleep. This is one reason why high-risk patients are not recommended for home-study monitoring.

The decision to perform any test, however, is made by your physician. Now that you have information about the methods available for evaluating snoring, you can discuss the relative pros and cons with your doctor.

Recommended Uses for Ambulatory Home Monitoring

1. As a screening test to determine if an overnight sleep study is indicated.

2. For the snorer whose history suggests a mild to moderate degree of sleep apnea without medical complications.

3. When a sleep disorders center is not available nearby.

4. As a follow-up study to test the effectiveness of medical or surgical treatment.

5. To measure the effectiveness of and calibrate for nasal continuous positive airway pressure treatment.

Tests for Hypersomnolence (Excessive Daytime Sleepiness)

The sleep disorders center also plays a vital role in diagnosing patients who suffer from excessive daytime sleepiness (EDS). We know that hypersomnolence is a frequent by-product of OSA and must be distinguished from other neurological conditions with similar symptoms, such as narcolepsy (an irresistible urge to fall asleep during the day).

If your medical history shows EDS and fatigue, you are likely to be scheduled for the Multiple Sleep Latency Test in the sleep disorders center. The standard sleep monitoring described earlier in this chapter is used to measure the time it takes to get back to sleep after being awakened. The patient is allowed to take four or five short naps at approximately 2-hour intervals during the day. He or she is monitored until stage 1 or 2 NREM sleep is reached or until 20 minutes have elapsed. Then he is awakened and the time it takes him to resume sleeping is recorded. The report contains the average sleep latency (the time taken to resume sleeping) as well as the number of REM periods during sleep.

This "nap test" allows the treating physician to grade the degree of hypersomnolence. Here is how physicians classify EDS:

Mild EDS: Patient can stay awake when motivated by work or social activities, but tends to become drowsy when external stimuli are removed.

Moderate EDS: Patient falls asleep when inactive or when at work, with increasing social and economic side effects as a result. Driving is a concern.

Severe EDS: Patient cannot stay awake during the day, even when motivated or stimulated. Such a patient tends to have a higher rate of industrial and automobile accidents.

After you spend a night in the sleep disorders center, or after an ambulatory study, your doctor will be able to determine just how severe your snoring is and whether any associated sleep apnea exists. At that point, you and he are ready to discuss treatment. However, before considering current methods that offer improvement or cure, I want to take a step back in time and examine some of the weird and wonderful devices and machines invented by would-be snore-stoppers during the last century.

CHAPTER 7

Snoring: The Mother of Invention

Snoring rattles so many households that the challenge to silence it has proven irresistible to inventors over the years. They have examined, poked, prodded, and analyzed this problem in search of a cure—any cure—that would bring nighttime silence to their bedrooms and overnight fame to themselves. Without a doubt, posterity would enshrine the inventor of a true snore-stopper. In fact, an article in a national health magazine once suggested that the Nobel committee should seriously consider awarding their peace prize to the person who would perfect a snoring cure!

Unfortunately, some would-be laureates have stumbled on their way to Stockholm. Consider this letter one man wrote to the *Ladies' Home Journal* in 1915.

Many years ago, I was one of those violent, house-shaking snorers, producing sounds like the rumbles of Mt. Etna. Suddenly a plan occurred to

*me, which, when adopted, effected a cure. Many
years have elapsed without any more snoring. My
only regret is that I have forgotten the plan!*

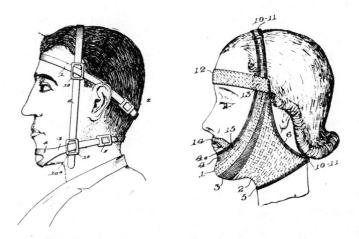

    A numbing variety of antisnoring devices have ap-
peared on the market, often listed in mail-order catalogs.
Many of these products have been enthusiastically pro-
moted and advertised, enjoying a season or two of popu-
larity before disappearing from view. And as farfetched as
many of these gadgets may appear, the concepts that in-
spire them are reasonably sound. All the inventors seem
to have had some understanding of the mechanics of snoring. This is evident from the fact that their devices can be
classified in the following categories:

- Appliances to keep the snorer off his back.
- Devices to keep the mouth closed and to
prevent the tongue from falling backward.
- Contrivances to extend the neck.
- Instruments to startle the snorer with a shock
or physical stimulus.

Peculiar Patents
That Seek to Cure

Over 300 of these antisnoring devices are listed in the gazettes of the U.S. Government Office of Patents. Perhaps, like so many inventions, they were born out of necessity, or even desperation. You would think that the disgruntled female snoree, prompted by all those sleepless nights she was forced to endure, would be the inventor. But no, virtually all the inventors are male.

It has long been observed that snoring is aggravated when the sleeper lies on his back. Ingenious minds eventually recognized that such snoring could be controlled by keeping the snorer on his side. As far back as the Revolutionary War, it was customary to sew a small cannonball into a pocket on the back of a soldier's uniform to keep him from sleeping on his back and awakening his comrades-in-arms with his snoring.

A turn-of-the-century version of this cannonball technique was developed by Leonidas Wilson in 1900. A leather brace wrapped around the snorer's upper body, holding a multipronged object between his shoulder

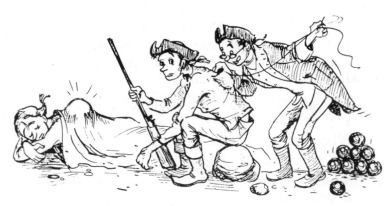

The invention of the first "snore ball."

blades—guaranteeing, I've no doubt, extreme discomfort if he should ever turn onto his back as he slept.

The modern version of this antisnoring technique is to sew a pocket on the back of a pajama top or T-shirt and

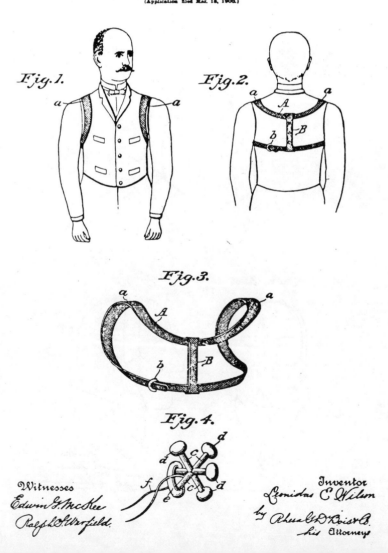

No. 663,825.

Patented Dec. 11, 1900.

L. E. WILSON.

SHOULDER BRACE AND ANTISNORING ATTACHMENT.

(Application filed Mar. 13, 1900.)

Fig. 1.

Fig. 2.

Fig. 3.

Fig. 4.

Witnesses
Edwin F. McKee
Ralph F. Warfield.

Inventor
Leonidas C. Wilson
by Rhea & D. Boisel Co.
his Attorneys

put a tennis ball or golf ball into it. Obviously, the sleeper experiences serious discomfort if he turns over onto his back, so he attempts to find a more comfortable position, ending his snoring in the process. Some sleepers, after several months of this conditioning technique, become so used to lying on their side that they can dispense with the snore-ball and sleep comfortably, snore-free.

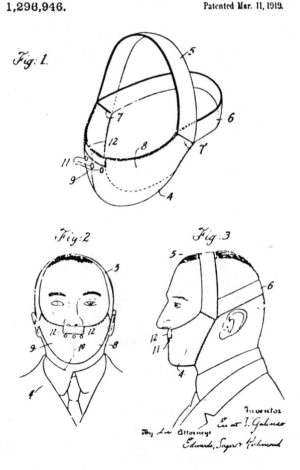

E. V. GALIARDO.
APPARATUS FOR CONTROLLING RESPIRATION.
APPLICATION FILED APR. 4, 1918.

1,296,946.

Patented Mar. 11, 1919.

Fig. 1.

Fig. 2.

Fig. 3.

Some motion-restraining devices are truly complex and ambitious, resembling a type of straitjacket that rigidly holds the snorer in one position on his side.

Many and varied inventions were created to restrict mouth breathing as a way to curb snoring. These products—called mouth-dams—follow the simple theory that if you breathe through your nose instead of your mouth, you won't snore.

In 1918, Ernest Galiardo developed and patented an elastic mask that fitted snugly over the sleeper's head, compressing his jaw so his mouth stayed closed. Galiardo called his creation an "apparatus for controlling respiration"—which it surely must have done!

Ten years later, Richard Garvey filed a patent for his mouth-closing device. It consisted of a blade that fit be-

Sept. 16, 1930.   R. GARVEY   1,775,718

MOUTH CLOSING DEVICE

Filed March 5, 1928

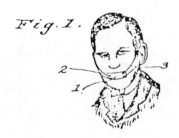

Fig. 1.

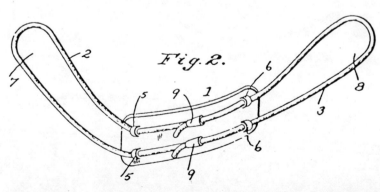

Fig. 2.

Feb. 3, 1953   E. L. LEPPICH   2,627,268
                              ANTISNORING DEVICE
                             Filed March 2, 1951

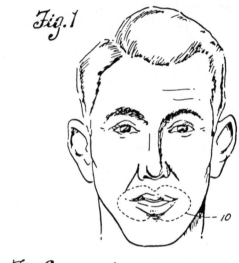

Fig.1

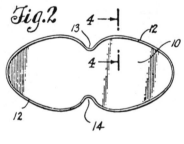

Fig.2

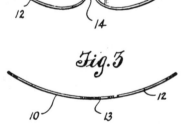

Fig.3

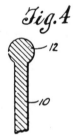

Fig.4

INVENTOR
ELSA L. LEPPICH
BY
Cook & Robinson
ATTORNEY

tween the snorer's lips, a guard to keep his mouth closed, and straps to secure the entire contraption to the sleeper's ears.

At last we come to a device invented by a woman. Elsa Leppich demonstrated to the world exactly how she felt about Mr. Leppich's rumblings when she patented her antisnoring device in 1951. It consisted of a tongue retainer and a lip guard. History does not record the success of the apparatus or the fate of the Leppich marriage. We can only hope for their happiness.

Chin Up, Chaps!

Other inventors endeavored to keep the snorer's mouth shut with a bewildering variety of chin straps and head caps. Antisnoring devices in this class represent some of the earliest inventions.

Way back in 1893, Francis W. Pulford of Carson, Michigan, filed a patent for a chin bandage which he called a facial molding device. Seven years later, Jacob S. Baughman of Burlington, Iowa, brought out a head bandage that included a chin sling with friction slides to facilitate movement.

I suspect, from the appearance of this device, that movement for the sleeper was somewhat of an impossible dream!

One patent that caught my attention as I was going through the files of old U.S. patent gazettes was an antimouth breathing device filed by John W. Rothenberger of Syracuse, Indiana, in 1919. I couldn't help wondering whether a snorer would be able to close his eyes and get one moment's rest when this contraption was in place.

I was also intrigued by the ingenuity of a mouth-

512,324. BANDAGE. Francis W. Pulford, Carson, Mich. Filed Apr. 17, 1893. Serial No. 470,605.

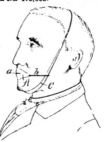

649,896. HEAD-BANDAGE. Jacob S. Baughman, Burlington, Iowa. Filed Jan. 4, 1900. Serial No. 373.

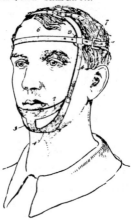

1,339,865. ANTI-MOUTH-BREATHING DEVICE. John W. Rothenberger, Syracuse, Ind. Filed May 29, 1919. Serial No. 300,574.

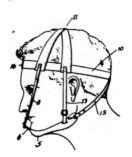

restraining device patented in 1948 by Cyrus Johnson. His invention offered the additional feature of keeping the upper airway expanded by extending the sleeper's neck. Although I fear that Johnson's appliance might have given many a snorer a stiff neck, the principle of keeping the airway open by elevating the chin is well recognized in modern medical practice.

2,528,370
DEVICE TO PREVENT MOUTH BREATHING
Cyrus H. Johnston, Richmond, Mo.
Application October 18, 1948, Serial No. 55,032

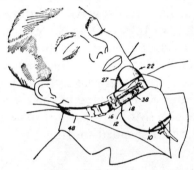

Johnson was actually anticipating an approach that was employed years later by Robert Elman, M.D., a St. Louis physician, in a clinical experiment he reported in the 1961 *Journal of the American Medical Association:*

> *A young patient wrote to me from his honeymoon, expressing fear that his marriage would fail because his snoring kept his bride awake so much that they were forced to occupy separate cabins. I had him examined and found no evidence of obstruction or disease in the nose or throat. Conventional treatment, such as making him sleep on his side and keeping his mouth closed, failed to bring relief and I therefore tried a new method. I remembered the obstructive breathing and snoring that frequently occurs during general anesthesia when*

*the chin is allowed to drop; this is relieved immedi-
ately by extending the neck. Acting on this idea, I
fitted the patient with a simple, easily applied and
removed orthopedic collar, asking him to use it at
night. He was greatly pleased, for the device had
eliminated his disability and for the first time his
wife had been able to get a good night's sleep. The
patient subsequently discarded the collar and
merely slept on his back with a small pillow at the
nape of his neck. He is now happily married and has
two children.*

Turning his attention to a different source of the
problem, Henry Molow, D. D. S., of Brooklyn, New York,
developed a nasal device which he called "the better
breathing tube." Fitting into the nose, this tube was designed to open the nasal passages and prevent collapse of
the soft tissues on each side of the nasal opening. Testi-
monials from Dr. Molow's patients using this device indicate that they all stopped snoring.

Crime and Punishment

As we know, the cannonball or snore-ball method
keeps the sleeper off his back through the principle of
reward and punishment. The success of this approach led
to the invention of modern devices aimed at changing
snorers' nightly behavior—conditioning them to become
blissfully quiet sleepers.

The Snore Stopper, currently sold by mail order,
claims to eliminate snoring "effectively and inexpen-
sively without drugs or surgery." A microphone in this
gadget picks up the sounds of snoring, triggering a mechanism which gives the sleeper a mild electric shock that is
not quite severe enough to awaken him. But the Snore
Stopper repeats the stimulus with each loud snore. The
object is, of course, to condition the snorer by making him

THE SNORE STOPPER
INSTRUCTION BOOKLET
Please read this instruction booklet before using the Snore Stopper.

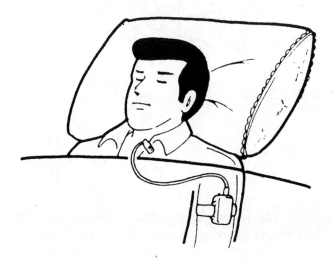

uncomfortable enough to change his behavior by electric shocks so he can enjoy a good night's rest without interruption.

One conditioning device, consisting of an electric detector that sets off a buzzer alarm in response to loud snoring, has a whimsical twist. The snorer has to get out of bed to deactivate the buzzer. The machine, however, provides a piece of candy as a reward.

A wonderful, though admittedly mischievous, Rube Goldberg-type device is the Snorgon 2000Z. As the blissful sleeper drifts deeper into unconsciousness, his body movements are monitored by a rumble sensor, and a blast-resistant microphone picks up the intensifying din

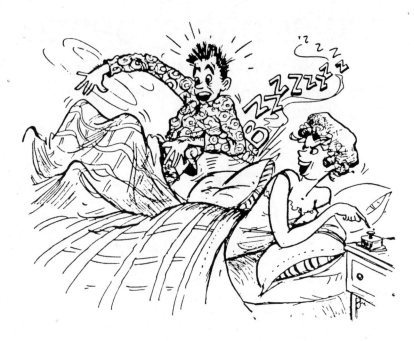

of his snoring. The readings continue while the snoring gets ever louder. At a critical point, the seismometer unleashes a series of snore deterrents upon the hapless snorer:

- A flashlight suddenly shines into his eyes.
- A "sound-activated beak tweeker" pinches him on the nose.
- A loudspeaker subjects him to the sound of his own ferocious snoring.
- A glass of cold water is tossed in his face.

Although the Snorgon 2000Z is clearly a tongue-in-cheek creation, some medical men were hard at work developing legitimate antisnore systems. Harvey Flack, M.D., of England, was one of these.

In 1960, Dr. Flack conducted experiments to determine what makes a snorer snore and what muscles, tis-

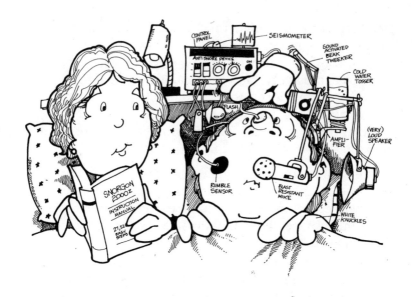

sues, and organs are involved. After establishing these facts, Dr. Flack and his colleagues developed a series of exercises, which they hoped would provide the long-sought-after cure for snoring. But these investigators knew their theory had to prove its value in practice. It had to be tested.

Snore No More with Dr. Flack

Dr. Flack put a notice in a British Medical Association magazine asking for snorers to volunteer for his project. The notice was headed, "Wanted Urgently—People Who Snore," and concluded with the promise: "There is at least an even chance that you will start the New Year with your snoring cured."

The response exceeded all expectations. Newspapers in Britain and countries all over the world reprinted the notices. Dr. Flack was deluged by letters and stopped counting after the first 3,000—even though the letters continued to pour in. Ultimately, 250 volunteer snorers were selected, representing a cross section of those whose jaws or tongues fell back during sleep or whose palates vibrated excessively. Dr. Flack and his medical team gave these volunteers a series of exercises that would tighten and improve the tone of their throat, jaw, and tongue muscles. Each volunteer was instructed to perform a set of exercises nightly for the next two weeks:

- Hold something, such as a pencil, firmly between your teeth for 10 minutes after going to bed but before settling down to sleep. After several minutes your jaw muscles will ache, and this is to be expected.
- For 2 to 3 minutes, press your fingers firmly against your chin and hold your jaw steady against the pressure of your fingers.
- Press your tongue against your lower teeth for 3 to 4 minutes. If you have no teeth, hold a finger to your mouth and press your tongue against it.

When the study was completed, Dr. Flack found that the exercises had been effective in many cases; in fact, the majority of the volunteers happily reported that their snoring had been appreciably curbed. Even so, Dr. Flack was less optimistic.

"I am not hopeful about a cure for snoring," he said. "It is true to say that if people are otherwise healthy and are throat snorers, about half can be helped if they work at the exercises. But otherwise it is unlikely that anyone will come up with anything dramatic or sensational.

"It comes to this: Snoring that threatens marriages or makes difficulties of that kind is in the province of the marriage counselor, not the doctor."

However, Dr. Flack's exercises appear to be safe and

may be worth trying, as they are designed to improve muscle tone in the tissues of the upper respiratory tract.

Safety Tips Concerning "Cures"

Not all patented methods for the cure of snoring are safe, and if you are going to experiment with any of them I recommend the following cautions:

- The use of any device that prevents mouth breathing requires that the user's nose be clear. Nasal obstruction of any cause—from colds, allergies, or polyps—may require medical or surgical treatment before using one of these appliances.
- Any body-restraining device can produce stiff joints and muscles and interfere with blood circulation.
- If you suspect that obstructive sleep apnea is associated with your snoring, seek medical advice rather than use over-the-counter "cures."
- Don't be fooled by expensive gadgets advertised as guaranteed cures in magazines and catalogs.
- Discuss any self-help device or method with your doctor to be sure it is reasonable for use in conjunction with your medical treatment.

We have examined the causes, effects, and complications of snoring. We have looked at antisnoring remedies and nostrums, available facilities, and appropriate physicians. Now we're ready to consider some of the more up-to-date approaches to this age-old problem.

CHAPTER 8

Modern Medical Treatment for Snoring

Wouldn't it be wonderful if every snorer's companion could go down to the local drugstore, purchase a bottle of "antisnore," sprinkle a few drops over her beloved's bedtime snack, and be rewarded with a silent, snore-free night?

Unfortunately, there is no such miracle product. But that doesn't mean snoring cannot be effectively curtailed or even cured. In fact, snoring can be alleviated by a variety of methods ranging from lifestyle changes to medical, mechanical, and surgical treatments. The method appropriate for you depends, to a large extent, on the answers to the following questions:

- Is my snoring loud enough to disturb my partner frequently?
- Is my snoring medically uncomplicated?
- If obstructive sleep apnea (OSA) accompanies my snoring, where does the obstruction occur in the upper respiratory tract?

- If OSA has been diagnosed during a sleep study, how severe is it? Has it progressed to the point of producing cardiovascular side effects?
- Do I suffer from excessive daytime sleepiness (EDS) in relation to the sleep apnea, and if so, to what degree?

Lifestyle Changes

If tests and observation prove that you do not suffer from sleep apnea, then a few simple changes in your lifestyle and sleep habits might reduce or possibly eliminate your snoring.

Where and how you sleep can affect your snoring. So can what you eat and drink, and when. And if you are overweight, that might be at the core of your snoring problem. Check your lifestyle against the tips and cautions below.

Sleep Habits

Changing your position during sleep is one possible answer to snoring, but not the only one. Consider these simple hints for a quiet, restful night's sleep.

- Sleep in a cool, well-ventilated room (ideal temperature 64° to 66°F).
- Eliminate intrusive sound and light from your bedroom so you won't be awakened accidentally.
- Listen to tapes of relaxing music or soothing natural sounds if you have trouble falling asleep.
- A glass of warm milk at bedtime can promote a restful night's sleep; it is rich in tryptophan, a

naturally occurring amino acid that acts as a mild sedative.

● Sleep on a firm mattress with a low pillow to keep your neck straight and reduce obstruction in your airway.

● If you snore only on your back, experimenting with various sleeping positions may bring snoring under control. One way is to start the night lying on your stomach, placing your arm under the pillow to steady your head. Another technique is to mold several cushions to each side of your body. If you can only sleep comfortably on your back, try sleeping without pillows to extend your head, or place a small pad under your chin to help keep your mouth closed.

● Sew a pocket between the shoulders of a pajama top or T-shirt and insert a golf or tennis ball. This is the snore-ball method, and though no clinical tests have been made of this technique, word of mouth confirms its success for some snorers.

Smoking

In my specialty of otolaryngology, we see the harmful effects of smoking on the tissues of the upper respiratory system. Smoking contributes to snoring by causing the following changes:

● Increased production of mucus in your nose and throat.

● Irritation and swelling of the mucous membranes of the throat and upper air passages.

● Lung irritation with increased bronchial secretions.

- Reduced oxygen uptake by the lungs.

I enthusiastically recommend that a snorer who smokes reduce or totally eliminate the habit as part of any self-help program to curb snoring.

Alcohol

All snorees can describe in colorful terms the exaggerated snoring and increased apneas that occur after their partner has been drinking. Alcohol is a central nervous system depressant that deepens the sleep level, increases muscle relaxation, and aggravates snoring.

- In a scientific study, a series of middle-aged men who seldom snored, began to do so after drinking substantial amounts of alcohol.

- Alcohol has produced apneas in heavy snorers who previously did not have this problem.

- A group of patients with mild OSA showed an increase in both frequency and severity of apneas (as recorded in a sleep lab) after consuming substantial amounts of alcohol.

- Alcohol tends to reduce muscle activity in the upper respiratory tract, making those muscles that stabilize the pharynx more prone to vibration and collapse.

- Alcohol depresses the arousal response in the breathing center of the brain stem by making it less sensitive to the chemical changes of reduced oxygen and increased carbon dioxide that accompany sleep apnea.

Based on our knowledge from these studies, we can offer the following advice to the snorer and snoree:

- Avoid the habit of an alcoholic nightcap before bed.
- Mild snorers should drink only in moderation.
- Heavy snorers and those with OSA should abstain from or drastically reduce their alcohol consumption.

Over-the-Counter Medications

Americans spend billions of dollars every year buying over-the-counter medications. Many of these drugs can be classified as central nervous system depressants whose effects on the brain are not too different from those of alcohol.

Medications such as cold cures, frequently taken in large doses during bouts of flu and colds, are often regarded by the public as completely safe and without side effects. Many, however, contain sedatives that can affect respiration and should be used with caution if you have any sleep-related breathing disorder.

As part of your treatment program, be sure to tell your physician if you are using any nasal sprays, aspirin, or other over-the-counter medications. Some of these may be exacerbating your snoring and might possibly be replaced by other treatments with fewer side effects.

Weight Loss

Though all the specific mechanisms have not yet been determined, obesity is known to increase snoring and apnea for the following reasons:

- The increased tissue bulk in the neck and throat of obese people, together with poor muscle tone, reduces the area of the upper air passage, making it more prone to obstruction.

- A large abdomen pressing on your diaphragm when you lie on your back increases the likelihood of OSA by further decreasing the size of your lungs and the amount of air you obtain with each breath.

While we cannot state the exact amount of weight loss that will benefit snorers and apnea sufferers, we do know that weight loss decreases and sometimes completely eliminates OSA.

- Sleep studies have demonstrated that a weight loss of 10 to 25 percent can eliminate apnea or significantly reduce the episodes.
- A study of markedly obese men who were over twice their ideal body weight showed a drop in the average number of apneas from 70 per hour to less than 10 per hour when they lost 30 to 60 percent of their original weight.

If you are overweight, it's clear that a weight-loss program is a *very* important step in your efforts to stop snoring. Nutrition counselors have developed some basic rules to follow:

- Know your facts as you count your calories. Be familiar with the percentages of fat, carbohydrates, and proteins in the foods you commonly eat. Learn about caloric values and read labels carefully. Attend classes at community hospitals where instruction on weight control is offered. Ask your doctor for brochures, booklets, or reference books that discuss nutrition, diet, and caloric values of foods.
- Develop calorie consciousness. Measure portions accurately and truthfully, replacing those

high-calorie foods now in your diet with foods of lower caloric value.

● Limit the fat calories in your diet to less than 30 percent of your total caloric intake each day.

● Try to avoid heavy meals at night. Eat your main meal during the day. And never eat to the point of feeling uncomfortable.

● Avoid fads. Watch out for diet pills and other gimmicks that are often advertised with a guarantee of easy, quick, surefire weight loss.

● Incorporate diet *and* exercise into your program. Regular exercise is an essential part of any weight-control plan. Dieting alone tends to focus on the lean muscle mass rather than the fat content of your body.

● Make judicious use of support groups and weight-loss programs supervised by qualified nutritionists, with the understanding that dieting is essentially a new way of life that calls for adopting healthier eating habits.

Admittedly, starting a diet and staying with it is not easy. For heavy snorers and those with apnea, it is particularly difficult, because sleep apnea sufferers experience repeated periods of oxygen starvation. Together with their hypersomnolence from sleep deprivation/ fragmentation, these snorers have low energy levels and this limits their ability to maintain a regular exercise schedule, often producing the vicious cycle shown on the opposite page.

If you are caught in this cycle, and are becoming discouraged in your efforts to diet and exercise, do not

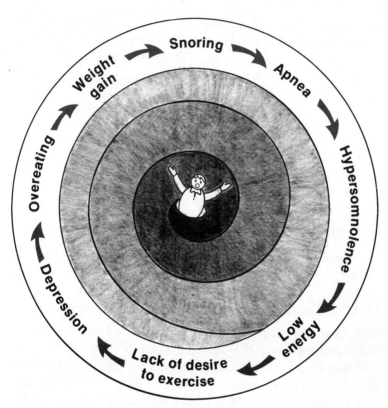

Snoring is part of the vicious cycle of impaired health.

lose hope. Later in this chapter I will discuss some options that provide encouragement and can help you break this pattern.

Drug Therapy

The medical profession is currently studying the use of drug therapy to treat snoring and OSA, but uniform success with any one drug has not been achieved. Some medications that theoretically showed benefits turned out to be disappointing in practice. Others have unpleasant, or even dangerous, side effects. But the field of drug therapy holds promise, and a number of medications have shown beneficial effects.

Medications currently prescribed include drugs that do the following:

- Open the nasal air passages.
- Stimulate respiration.
- Promote wakefulness.
- Inhibit the rapid eye movement (REM) sleep stage.

Let's consider each group of medications—when they're indicated, their benefits, and their side effects.

Drugs That Open the Nasal Air Passages

As we have seen, nasal congestion can cause or aggravate snoring. Over-the-counter nasal decongestant drops and sprays may clear your nasal passages and allow you to breathe more easily for a while, but they also contribute to a phenomenon known as the rebound effect. It works this way: The chemicals in nose drops that relieve congestion do so by constricting the nasal blood vessels and shrinking the mucous membranes. Shortly after application, however, the vessels expand again and the mucous membranes begin to swell. With repeated use, the membranes lose their ability to react and may remain in a permanently swollen, congested state. Let me share my impressions of some other commonly used products.

Simple saline sprays can moisten mucous membranes. These sprays are widely available and contain nothing more than salt water. They have no ill effects on the nasal mucous membranes. A word of caution here: Don't make your own spray. It's tempting to add a few teaspoons of salt to a bottle of water and make up your own formula, but I recommend against it. Purchase the commercial nasal saline sprays because they contain the same proportion of salt to water as your body's blood plasma has. If you should put too much salt in your home-made remedy, it might burn your nose or interfere with the desired moisturizing effect of the solution.

A new type of nosedrop called phosphocholanamin (derived from lecithin, a natural substance found in soy beans and other foods) works to reduce snoring by lubricating the nasal passages. In a clinical trial of these drops at the University of Toronto Sleep Clinic, nearly half the subjects experienced a reduced frequency and intensity of their snoring. Although it appears to be safe, this drug has not yet received Food and Drug Administration (FDA) approval.

Synthetic cortisone nasal sprays prescribed for allergies have proven extremely valuable in treating not only seasonal hay fever and perennial nasal allergy, but also in reducing the snoring that often accompanies the increased congestion. In my opinion, they are simple and safe to use. Clinical studies show none of the side effects seen with taking systemic cortisone medications. These nasal medications, however, must be prescribed by a physician.

Drugs That Stimulate Respiration

Many of the drugs used to treat lung conditions, such as asthma, have also been suggested for snoring and OSA.

Progesterone. During pregnancy and certain phases of the menstrual cycle, a woman's rate and depth of breathing increases. Researchers have been able to produce a similar respiratory effect in males by giving them progesterone (a female sex hormone). For that reason, this drug has been used to manage a certain type of sleep apnea in heavy snorers. In theory it works by stimulating the respiratory center in the brain and by redistributing body fat.

Indications: Progesterone has been most successful in treating overweight, severe snorers with predominantly central apnea.

Side effects: Hair loss, impotence, and reduced sex drive. These effects usually stop when the drug is discontinued. They can also be reversed if male hormones are administered. A distinct drawback of this hormone is its tendency to produce uterine bleeding in postmenopausal females and to aggravate growths of the prostate gland in elderly males. Progesterone should not be used in patients who have a history of liver disease or blood-clotting disorders.

Acetazolamide. This drug acts on the kidneys and stimulates respiration by increasing the acidity in the blood. This chemical change is known as metabolic acidosis.

Indications: This drug has been used in some cases of central apnea with occasional beneficial effects. However, there are no reports of its successful use in treating OSA.

Side effects: Numbness, tingling in the hands and feet, drowsiness, and confusion. This drug should not be used if there is a history of liver or kidney disease.

Theophylline. This drug, frequently used for asthma, stimulates breathing by sensitizing the respiratory center in the brain stem to the stimulating effects of carbon dioxide.

Indications: Theophylline has not shown much promise in treating OSA, but appears to be of some benefit in treating central apnea.

Side effects: Nausea, irritability, and cardiac arrhythmias.

Drugs That Promote Wakefulness

Amphetamines. Although they have no direct effect on OSA, such stimulants can provide symptomatic relief from excessive daytime sleepiness (EDS). They can be prescribed for short periods when other medical therapies are unsuccessful and for patients who refuse any type of mechanical or surgical treatment. The side effects to look for include anxiety, agitation, insomnia, and weight loss. Of course, amphetamines are addictive and can be abused.

Drugs That Inhibit the REM Sleep Stage

Because most severe snoring and OSA occur during REM sleep, a drug that can shorten this phase of the sleep cycle can also diminish the incidence of apnea.

Protriptyline. The most commonly prescribed drug for sleep apnea associated with daytime sleepiness, it works by inhibiting REM sleep, that stage during which most apneas occur.

Indications: Protriptyline can be used for snorers with mild to moderate OSA who suffer from EDS.

Side effects: Dry mouth, urinary retention, and cardiac arrhythmias. This drug can increase muscle movement (especially leg movement) during sleep. It should not be used by patients over 60 years of age, those who are overweight, or those who have any psychological or emotional disorders.

Mouth Devices to Improve the Upper Airway

What if the lifestyle changes and medications described above as measures against snoring and apnea are not suitable or do not work for you? A number of orthodontic and mechanical devices are available that might prove beneficial.

In 1980, Rosalind Cartwright, Ph.D., and Charles Samuelson, M.D., of Chicago, Illinois, introduced a tongue-retaining device as an aid for patients who suffered from sleep-induced upper airway obstruction. Made of a soft plastic material that attaches to the tongue by suction, this device pulls the tongue forward and widens the pharyngeal airway at the same time. Severe snorers and mild to moderate apnea sufferers can learn to sleep with the device in place for 3 to 4 hours per night. However, discomfort or eventual loss of suction prevents the wearer from using it longer than that.

This appliance is sometimes recommended for severe snorers and for patients with OSA who cannot tolerate other treatments and refuse to have any type of corrective surgery. The results of a clinical trial, published in 1982, showed that the device substantially reduced snoring and the number and duration of apneas. More than half of the patients in this trial also reported relief from their daytime sleepiness.

Not surprisingly, some patients simply cannot tolerate sleeping with a foreign device in their mouth. It makes some of them gag and drool. If you decide to try it, you should be examined by an otolaryngologist first to be sure you have a clear nasal airway, because the tongue-retaining device blocks your mouth. Medical attention, even surgery, may be required to ensure that your nasal passages are clear before using this mouth device and the others described in this section.

Among the antisnoring mouth protheses that have become available in recent years, some are relatively easy to apply, while others require multiple fittings by a dentist or orthodontist. They all fit firmly over the teeth and expand the pharyngeal airway by advancing the jaw bone.

One innovative appliance called an oral medical device has the combined functions of lifting the soft palate, equalizing air pressure in the oropharynx, and keeping the jaw in a forward position. This device is among the few to gain FDA approval and, in clinical trials, it has been beneficial to more than 50 percent of patients treated with it for snoring and sleep apnea.

An orthotic device developed at the University of New Mexico by Wolfgang W. Schmidt-Nowara, M.D., and Thomas Meade, D.D.S., shows a great deal of promise. The device can be fitted by any trained dentist and most wearers say that they can wear it comfortably throughout the night. Of the severe snorers with mild to moderate sleep apnea who used it in a clinical trial, 80 percent were successful in curbing their apnea and reducing EDS. Most claimed that their snoring was diminished or eliminated.

Prosthetic appliances are valuable indicators when surgery is being considered. If they help, then surgery is likely to help, too. These devices are also useful for patients whose general health makes surgery inadvisable, and for those who have had upper airway surgery with limited success.

If you are considering a mouth sleep device, here are my recommendations:

Have a complete sleep study and upper airway examination. Then talk with your physician about whether a mouth device is appropriate for you.

Get a proper fit. Mouth devices are usually fitted by orthodontists or dentists trained in this technique, so your regular physician may not be familiar with them. However, the medical director of your local sleep disorders center should know about these prostheses and be able to recommend a suitable practitioner for you.

Ask about the cost. Some devices are relatively simple and require no more than one or two visits to the dentist and several X-rays of the head before fitting. Others, which require multiple orthodontic visits and many X-rays, can prove to be quite expensive.

Keep an open mind. Understand that there will be some initial discomfort while wearing an orthotic device and that a learning period is necessary before you can use it comfortably.

Be honest with your physician. These devices were never expected to cure every case of apnea. If, after a trial period, the device still gags you and disturbs your sleep, or if it does not appear to help your snoring and apnea symptoms, feel free to say so and discuss other options of treatment.

Nasal Continuous Positive Airway Pressure

In 1981, Colin Sullivan, M.D., of the University of Sydney, Australia, described a method that eliminated upper airway collapse by using a pump to provide a constant air pressure into the pharynx during sleep. Called nasal continuous positive airway pressure (Nasal CPAP; pronounced "see-pap"), this pump generates enough pressure in the collapsible part of the upper airway to hold the tissues apart and inhibit their tendency to occlude during the relaxed phases of sleep. This technique is known as pneumatic splinting.

Recommended for severe snorers and those who have been diagnosed as suffering from any degree of OSA, Nasal CPAP is being prescribed with increasing enthusiasm because of its high level of success in treating sleep-related breathing disorders.

Resembling a small computer terminal in size, the Nasal CPAP systems currently available weigh 9 to

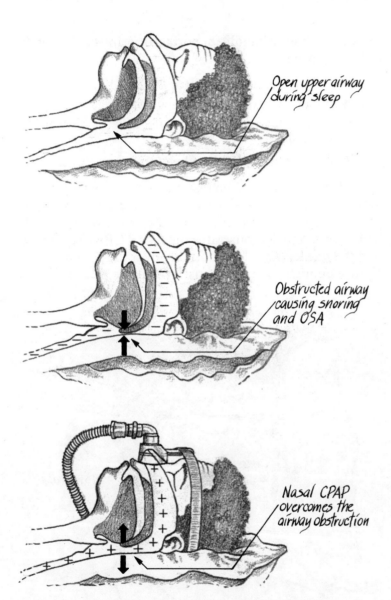

Open upper airway during sleep

Obstructed airway causing snoring and OSA

Nasal CPAP overcomes the airway obstruction

The top illustration shows a normal airway. The middle shows the obstructed airway (note arrows). Nasal continuous positive airway pressure (Nasal CPAP) increases air pressure going into the nose, eliminating the obstruction (see arrows in bottom illustration).

18 pounds, have a handle for portability, and consist of the following parts:

- An air pressure generator called a blower.
- A closely fitting nasal mask with head straps.
- A flexible tube or hose connecting the blower to the mask.
- A valve assembly to adjust air pressure.

After the initial sleep test, the patient usually spends another night in the sleep disorders center with all the sensors applied just as they would be for a regular study. The technician demonstrates the Nasal CPAP equipment and the mask is fitted comfortably over the patient's nose, tightly enough to prevent any air leakage. Made of a soft

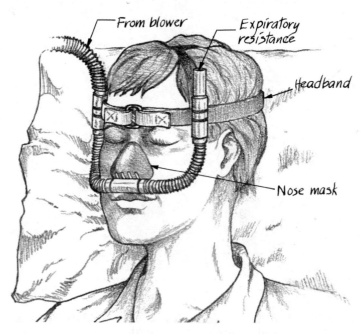

From blower

Expiratory resistance

Headband

Nose mask

The nasal continuous positive airway pressure (Nasal CPAP) mask is comfortable enough to allow for a full night's sleep.

material, usually molded silicon, the mask creates a tight fit without undue irritation.

Once the patient falls asleep, the lab technician slowly adjusts the valve on the blower unit, gradually increasing the air pressure going into the snorer's nose until the apneas are eliminated. The patient then sleeps comfortably throughout the night and the technician makes periodic checks to ensure that apneas are not recurring.

In the morning, if the patient feels that he had a refreshing night's sleep and wishes to try Nasal CPAP at home, he can purchase a unit or obtain one on a monthly rental basis from a medical supply company specializing in home respiratory equipment. In successful cases, the patient's EDS usually disappears within a matter of days. He is able to return to the physical and mental activities that were diminished by his sleep apnea. In some cases where the initial response was good, a lab technician may have to readjust the valve pressure if the apneas recur or if the EDS returns.

Though the initial fitting and adjustment for Nasal CPAP is commonly conducted in a sleep disorders center, it can also be done in the patient's home by a qualified technician using portable monitoring equipment.

Nasal CPAP has proved effective for approximately 85 percent of all OSA sufferers. In the majority of cases the apneas are eliminated, snoring is silenced, and the patient and his partner can sleep without interruption.

Patients who can benefit from Nasal CPAP include the following:

- Severe snorers in whom changes in lifestyle, including weight loss, have failed to curtail snoring.
- Snorers who display symptoms of EDS.
- Those with severe snoring and apnea who are

candidates for surgery, but who wish to try a less invasive type of treatment first.

● Victims of the sleep apnea syndrome who are having difficulty losing weight in preparation for surgery, because of the vicious cycle described earlier.

● Those recovering from surgery. The positive pressure produced by the Nasal CPAP can over-

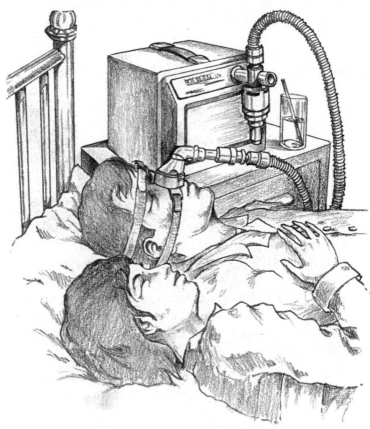

Bringing nasal continuous positive airway pressure (Nasal CPAP) into the bedroom means *both* of you can sleep.

come any airway obstruction caused by postoperative swelling after surgery on the throat and jaws. Nasal CPAP can also be of great value in reducing the risks of postoperative respiratory failure that can arise from anesthesia and the use of pain medications and sedatives.

● People whose sleep studies show the presence of central apnea when, in fact, they have either mixed apnea or OSA. Patients in this group are now described as suffering from central-like apnea, and are referred to as positive Nasal CPAP responders.

● Those whose EDS might be caused by either sleep apnea or narcolepsy may have the diagnosis resolved through the use of Nasal CPAP. The hypersomnolence of OSA will usually improve with Nasal CPAP, while the symptoms of narcolepsy will continue despite this treatment.

Useful as it is, not everyone can or wants to use Nasal CPAP. Here are some of the disadvantages:

● From 15 to 20 percent of patients cannot tolerate wearing the mask during sleep. They report feelings of claustrophobia and suffocation.

● Some patients complain of dry mouth and nose, sore throat, eye irritation, and ear infections.

● The noise of the pump can be disturbing to the bedroom partner. (This situation should soon be eliminated with improved technology.)

● Some women report an initial loss of romantic feelings while sharing a bed with a partner

wearing a device that resembles a scuba mask.
(This is usually overcome as the snorer regains
his general health and his snoring is eliminated.)
● There is no *cure.* The sleep apnea symptoms,
together with snoring, recur rapidly when the
use of the pump is discontinued.
● The Nasal CPAP is an additional piece of baggage to carry with you when you travel.

For those patients who cannot tolerate Nasal CPAP, a
new refinement called Biphasic Nasal CPAP (BiPAP™)
appears to hold much promise. Unlike CPAP, which exerts a gentle constant pressure through the nose during
both inhalation and exhalation, the BiPAP device allows
the physician to reduce the air pressure for the exhalation
phase. This lowers the resistance against which the patient has to breathe out. The BiPAP machine can simultaneously be adjusted to breathe at a particular frequency, a
feature that is of value for those patients whose breathing
is compromised by disorders of muscle weakness such as
muscular dystrophy or multiple sclerosis. In addition,
BiPAP should be beneficial for snorers and apnea sufferers
who are markedly obese.

Experimental prototypes have been tested with success in leading sleep disorders clinics and this device is
now available. Simultaneous to these developments is
the introduction of electronic pacemakers, which stimulate the muscles that keep the upper airway open. Similar
to cardiac pacemakers, these devices are triggered by the
severe snoring and apnea that follow a sudden decrease in
the size of the airway.

Nasal CPAP, which is available throughout the country, now plays a most valuable role in the treatment of
snorers with established sleep apnea, especially where

their daytime sleepiness is becoming troublesome. Admittedly, these devices require some getting used to, but patients who persevere usually obtain immediate improvement in their symptoms.

For many, however, such perseverance is not always practical or possible. For this reason, surgical methods are the next treatment options to consider in order to silence snorers and bring some rest to their disturbed nights.

Surgery for Snorers

Although physicians recognized long ago that the uvula and soft palate were the culprits causing the vibrating noise of snoring, early attempts to excise these offending organs or stiffen them with chemical injections were not very effective. These early failures no doubt contributed to the public's conviction that snoring was an irreversible nuisance, and set back the attempts of physicians who sought a surgical cure.

Modern surgical treatment to relieve snoring was started in Japan in 1952 by Takenosuke Ikematsu, M.D. A young woman whose marriage was suffering because of her extremely loud snoring was cured of her problem by removing excess tissue from the back of her throat. Inspired by his success, Dr. Ikematsu recorded and studied the snoring of over 300 patients during the next four years. He continued to perform these surgeries and reported his results in the medical literature, claiming a success rate of over 80 percent. The procedures Dr. Ikematsu developed, which he called palatectomy and partial uvulectomy, consisted of excising excess tissue of the soft palate together with part of the uvula.

The groundwork established by this insightful surgeon set the stage for a procedure introduced into the United States in 1980 by Shiro Fujita, M.D., at the Henry Ford Hospital in Detroit, Michigan. His operation, called uvulopalatopharyngoplasty—which, according to some surgeons, is easier to perform than pronounce—consists of enlarging the patient's throat passage by removing the uvula, tonsils, and part of the soft palate. Abbreviated UPPP, Dr. Fujita's surgery is today the most commonly performed procedure for severe snoring and OSA.

Similar surgical techniques, also based on Dr. Ikematsu's work, were being developed at the same time by F. Blair Simmons, M.D., at Stanford University Medical School. He and Dr. Fujita taught UPPP techniques to surgeons in this country and published papers on the procedure and its success. Their efforts have led to courses and seminars—often presented by sleep disorders centers—where surgeons are instructed in UPPP procedures, the determination of criteria for this surgery, and methods for standardizing postoperative results.

A single operation certainly cannot do the job for all snorers, as obstructions may occur in different areas of the upper airway, some requiring more than one surgery. If a patient needs multiple surgeries—called revision of the upper airway—these may be in stages or performed in one session, depending on the scope of the procedures and the attitude of the individual surgeon.

The philosophy of these surgeries on the upper airway is to eliminate snoring and, ideally, all symptoms of OSA, without interfering with the patient's basic functions of speech, breathing, and swallowing.

The decision to have surgery is obviously a major one and should not be considered until after you have done the following:

- Undergone a thorough medical evaluation including an examination of the upper respiratory tract by an otolaryngologist.
- Had an overnight sleep study.
- Received a detailed explanation from your

physician regarding all of the various options of treatment available to you.

● Tried lifestyle changes (including weight loss) and discussed noninvasive approaches (medications, a mouth device, or Nasal CPAP) with your physician.

If snoring continues to disrupt your life despite these measures, or your health is still affected by such symptoms of apnea as EDS, you should talk with your physician about surgical treatment. The surgeries you discuss will come under five headings, corresponding to the anatomical area of the operation. They are:

● The nasal cavity (the nose and nearby structures).

● The nasopharynx (the area behind the nose).

● The oropharynx (the throat and nearby structures).

● The hypopharynx (the area behind and below the jaw).

● The trachea (the windpipe).

Surgery on the Nasal Cavity

Surgical operation: Nasal septoplasty

Definition: An operation to improve the nasal airway by realigning the bone and cartilage separating the two sides of the nose.

Indications: This surgery is recommended if you snore severely, have not responded to conservative treatment, and it has been determined that airway obstruction is caused by a deviated nasal septum.

Postoperative care: You will probably go home on the same day as the surgery. Nasal packing is removed by the

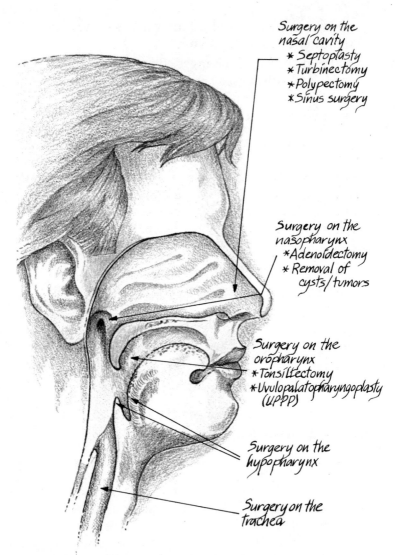

Surgery on the
nasal cavity
  * Septoplasty
  * Turbinectomy
  * Polypectomy
  * Sinus surgery

Surgery on the
nasopharynx
  * Adenoidectomy
  * Removal of
    cysts/tumors

Surgery on the
oropharynx
  * Tonsillectomy
  * Uvulopalatopharyngoplasty
    (UPPP)

Surgery on the
hypopharynx

Surgery on the
trachea

Surgical measures for snoring and sleep apnea.

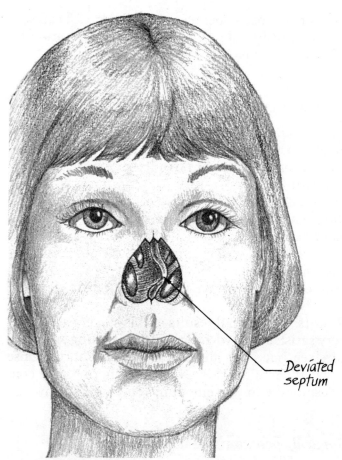

Deviated
septum

A deviated nasal septum.

surgeon within a day or two. For about one week after surgery, your nose will be congested, though by this time you will have already resumed your normal activities.

Results: Although nasal septoplasty is usually successful in clearing the nasal airway, it is not always effective in eliminating snoring. If you continue to snore following this operation, there may be some other obstructive site in your upper respiratory tract, and you will most likely be advised to undergo further evaluation by your physician and have an overnight sleep study.

Surgical operation: Turbinectomy

Definition: An operation to reduce the size of the turbinate bones that lie along the inner walls of the nose and have become enlarged from allergy or infection.

Indications: This surgery is recommended if your snoring is associated with severe chronic nasal obstruction from enlarged turbinates that does not respond to medical treatment.

Postoperative care: Postoperative care for turbinectomy is similar to that of nasal septoplasty, though more frequent follow-up visits are usually required to clean the nasal cavities.

Results: The overall results of this surgery are generally very satisfactory, with improved breathing and more restful sleep once the mucous membranes in the nose have healed. Here too, however, your snoring may continue despite the improvement in your nasal airway.

Surgical operation: Nasal polypectomy

Definition: An operation to remove polyps from the nose and sinuses.

Indications: This surgery is recommended if your snoring is caused by nasal obstruction or chronic sinus infection from nasal polyps. These waterlogged swellings develop in the mucous membrane lining of the nose and sinuses as a result of allergy or infection. Blocked sinuses are frequently treated at the same time. Viewing the inside of the nose through a rigid endoscope (or telescope) and using specially designed surgical instruments, the

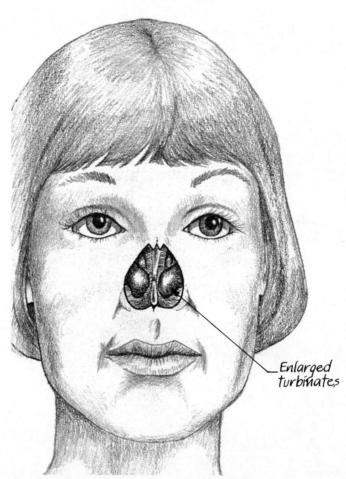

Nasal obstruction from turbinate enlargement.

surgeon removes polyps from the sinuses, establishing natural drainage and restoring sinus function. Before surgery is considered, you should have allergy tests, if appropriate, and medical treatment—which may include allergy shots or steroid nasal sprays.

Postoperative care: The care required after this surgery is similar to that of the previous surgeries. Because

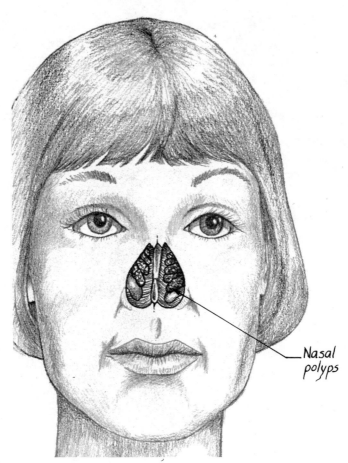

Nasal polyps.

nasal polyps tend to recur, however, you will probably be asked by your physician to make periodic follow-up visits, combined with some form of anti-allergic control.

Results: Nasal polypectomy usually produces gratifying results, allowing the patient's return to normal nasal breathing. If your snoring is directly due to nasal obstruction, improvement should occur once the passage is clear.

Surgery on the Nasopharynx

Surgical operation: Adenoidectomy

Definition: A surgical procedure to remove the spongey lymphoid tissue from the back of the nose.

Indications: Adenoidectomy is recommended for children with severe snoring, nasal obstruction, and constant mouth breathing due to enlarged adenoids. This surgery is considered only when all medical measures have failed and other causes of nasal congestion, including allergies, have been excluded.

Postoperative care: Other than a mild sore throat, the

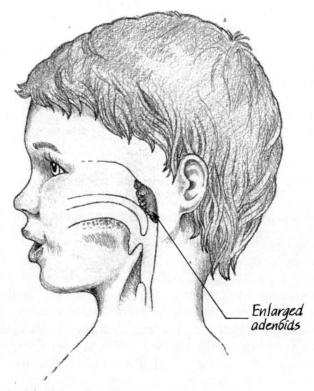

Enlarged
adenoids

Obstructed postnasal airway before adenoidectomy.

recovery tends to be quick and the child is usually back to normal activities within a day or two.

Results: This procedure is highly successful, and the child's snoring, mouth breathing, nasal obstruction, and apnea, customarily disappear within days of the surgery.

Surgical operation: Removal of nasopharyngeal masses

Definition: Surgical removal of polyps, cysts, or swellings from the back of the nose.

Indications: When it has been determined that snoring occurs due to obstructions in the nasopharynx.

Postoperative care: Varies according to the source of the swelling and scope of the surgery performed. In most cases, recovery is rapid, with minimal discomfort, and normal activities are resumed within a few days.

Results: Snoring usually stops after the nasal airway has been cleared, if this obstruction is the predominant cause.

Surgery of the Oropharynx

Surgical operation: Tonsillectomy (in children)

Definition: Surgical removal of the tonsils

Indications: Tonsillectomy for snoring in childhood is recommended when the child's snoring is severe and is accompanied by constant mouth breathing, frequent colds, and restless sleeping; all attributed to enlarged tonsils. Often combined with adenoidectomy, removal of a child's tonsils is only advised when the symptoms of severe upper respiratory obstruction persist despite thorough medical treatment.

Postoperative care: The child will have a sore throat, usually lasting four to six days, responding to pain medication, ample tender loving care, and the traditional rewards of ice cream, Jell-O, Popsicles, and milkshakes.

Results: Snoring and apnea usually disappear shortly after surgery.

Surgical operation: Tonsillectomy (in adults)

Definition: Surgical removal of tonsils

Indications: Tonsillectomy for adults is performed for the same reasons as in childhood. Other anatomical changes, such as an elongated uvula, however, may be contributing to snoring and obstructive sleep apnea (OSA) in adults, and additional surgery may be advised—the most frequent being UPPP.

Postoperative care: Adults do not recover quite as quickly as children, and can experience a painful throat

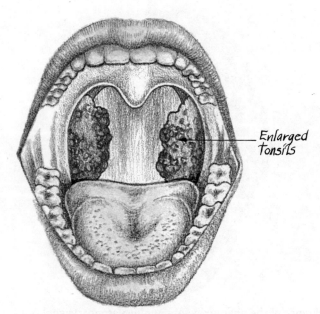

Enlarged
Tonsils

Large tonsils obstructing the air passage of the throat.

for seven to ten days—requiring rest, medication, and supportive care.

Results: Tonsillectomy alone may not cure an adult's snoring, and for this reason the following procedure is often performed at the same time.

Surgical operation: Uvulopalatopharyngoplasty (UPPP)

Definition: An operation to enlarge the throat. By removing the tonsils, if they are still present, together with the uvula and edge of the soft palate, the surgeon expands the airway, making the oropharynx resistant to collapse and excess vibration. This operation has aptly been termed a *face-lift on the back of the throat.*

Indications: If you are a severe snorer with an Apnea Index (see page 97) of more than 15 or 20 and oxygen desaturation below 85 percent, most surgeons now agree

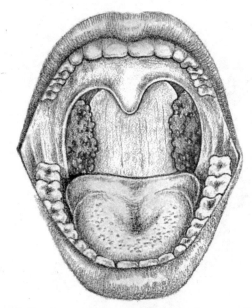

Appearance of the pharynx before uvulopalatopharyngoplasty (UPPP), an operation to enlarge the throat.

that you can benefit from UPPP, after all conservative methods of treatment have failed. In addition, UPPP is recommended if there is an obstruction at the back of your throat causing apnea—regardless of the severity—and you suffer from hypersomnolence. UPPP for snoring without apnea is only considered when a patient's snoring is severe enough to threaten the intimacy of a relationship; that is, when a couple can no longer sleep in the same room, and all other approaches have failed.

Postoperative care: Patients with severe degrees of OSA or those who are very obese may require a temporary tracheostomy prior to surgery to protect their upper airway. For the same reason, nasal continuous positive airway pressure (Nasal CPAP) and careful monitoring are often advised during the first few postoperative days. Patients have a very sore throat for at least seven to ten days following this surgery, and will remain hospitalized for several days until the pain subsides and they are able to swallow comfortably.

Results: The success rate for eliminating snoring or substantially reducing it is about 95 percent. However, experts disagree on the exact criteria for determining the surgical success of UPPP for OSA. When sleep apnea is present, *complete* success is judged by the elimination of apneas, a return to normal oxygen saturation levels, and the absence of EDS. The debate regarding UPPP revolves around whether or not the persistence of *any* symptoms of OSA after surgery can qualify the procedure as being fully successful. To clarify this issue, a postoperative sleep study is always recommended for patients who have had UPPP for OSA.

It's important to note some of the side effects of UPPP. In some cases regurgitation of fluids through the nose and a nasal quality to the voice can occur for several weeks following the surgery. These events are usually temporary and disappear once the postoperative swelling subsides.

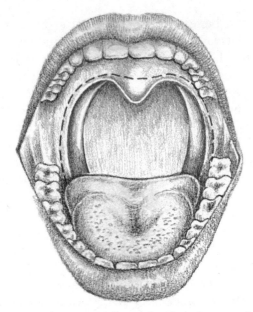

Appearance of the pharynx before uvulopalatopharyngoplasty (UPPP): The tonsils have been removed and the dotted line indicates where the uvula and the edge of the soft palate will be trimmed.

If your doctor recommends UPPP, check to see whether it is covered by your insurance policy. Payment is sometimes denied when the operation is performed for snoring alone.

Surgery on the Hypopharynx

For some patients who have had a UPPP operation, symptoms of OSA may persist. As a result, surgeons have developed a series of more complex surgical procedures. These surgeries are never done for snoring alone. Instead they are restricted to that small percentage of patients—most of whom suffer from marked obesity—whose airway is still blocked because of a recessed jaw or a bulky tongue intruding into the back of their throat. Some of these procedures include midline partial glossectomy (reduction of the tongue), mandibular osteotomy with hyoid suspension and tongue advancement (elevation of throat muscles and repositioning of the tongue), and maxillary and mandibular advancement (realignment of upper and lower jaws).

These surgeries are infrequently performed and are done by a relatively small number of highly specialized surgeons working in conjunction with sleep disorders centers. Should you be a candidate for such surgery, I recommend that you discuss the procedure in detail with your physician, recognizing that these operations are indicated only for incapacitating sleep apnea, when all other methods of treatment have failed.

Surgery on the Trachea

Surgical operation: Tracheostomy

Definition: A surgical procedure for opening the trachea (windpipe) in order to bypass the upper airway.

Indications: Until the early 1980s, tracheostomy was the accepted surgical treatment—the only one available—for severe OSA, especially in obese patients, before the development of UPPP and surgery on the hypopharynx. Today, tracheostomy is rarely done as a primary procedure and is never done for snoring alone. Instead, it may be an emergency procedure for severely apneic patients with life-threatening cardiac arrhythmias or airway obstruction. In addition, tracheostomy to protect the airway may be required prior to performing UPPP in obese patients with severe forms of apnea. This operation may also be done as an adjunct to hypopharyngeal surgeries for similar reasons.

Postoperative care: Tracheostomy requires intensive postoperative care. Accumulated secretions from the lungs have to be suctioned through the tracheostomy tube; inhaled air must be artificially humidified because the tracheostomy bypasses the natural airway.

Results: A tracheostomy immediately relieves all the symptoms of OSA. However, living with a tube in your throat presents serious difficulties. You have to cover the tube in order to speak; there are always increased secretions; there is an added tendency toward lung infections, and you are not permitted to swim. For these reasons, once the tracheostomy has bypassed the upper airway obstruction, today surgeons perform a subsequent operation, if possible, in an effort to cure the OSA permanently, remove the tracheostomy tube, and allow the patient to resume a normal life.

Deciding on Surgery

Discuss any recommended surgery with your physician, keeping in mind that the preceding descriptions are not meant to be definitive but introductory—familiarizing you with some of the basic surgeries being practiced today in the treatment of snoring and OSA. Ask your physician about his or her experience with these surgeries, and about the exact nature of the procedure being performed, possible complications, length of time in the hospital, loss of time from work, and any other questions relevant to your concerns. Of course, your questions should also deal with the cost of surgery and whether it will be covered by your insurance, recognizing that in addition to your surgeon's fee there will be other expenses—the hospital's charges and the anesthesiologist's fees.

The decision to undergo surgery should not be taken lightly. Like any other decision it should be made *only* after you have obtained a body of well-balanced information on the subject.

You must feel satisfied that objective research and good sense point to surgery as the best possible solution to your problem. Only then should you feel free to take such a step.

Here's to Quiet Nights from Now On

We have come a long way together in our discussion of snoring, and I hope this book has provided you with the confidence that snoring need not be a permanent condition that affects your life and your relationships. Modern medical approaches have developed to the point where sufferers can be cured, their lives returned to normal, and their relationships, to happiness.

This does not always mean that their snoring is completely eliminated, however, and I want to be candid about this. In some instances, a person will continue to snore, despite treatment, but usually at considerably lower levels and without producing the disturbance and conflict that previously threatened his relationships and life. Wives can return to the bedroom and snorers can resume being husbands.

It is my wish that your efforts in pursuit of a cure will bring vigor to your days and silence to your nights. In the words of David Frishberg, a well-known songwriter and jazz entertainer:

> I don't need no vitamins or tonics
> Or hormones off some monkey in the trees
> I don't need no high or low colonics
> Or jelly from royal honeybees
> I got to get me some zzzzs.
>
> I don't want no whiskey or no highballs
> I don't need no headaches or d.t.'s
> Just dig these satchels underneath my
>   eyeballs
> Now if I'm going to get rid of these
> I better get me some zzzzs.

G-O-O-O-D NIGHT!

Sleep Disorders Centers

United States

This roster of member centers, accredited by the American Sleep Disorders Association, was compiled on October 1, 1989. For further information and an updated list contact:

American Sleep Disorders Association
604 Second Street SW
Rochester, MN 55902
(507) 287-6006

Alabama

Sleep Disorders Center of Alabama
Affiliated with Baptist Medical
  Center Montclair
800 Montclair Road
Birmingham, AL 35213
(205) 592-5650

Sleep Disorders Laboratory
The Children's Hospital of Alabama
1600 Seventh Avenue South
Birmingham, AL 35233
(205) 939-9386

Sleep-Wake Disorders Center
University of Alabama
University Station
Birmingham, AL 35294
(205) 934-7110

North Alabama Sleep
  Disorders Center
Huntsville Hospital
101 Sivley Road
Huntsville, AL 35801
(205) 533-8553

Sleep Disorders Center
Mobile Infirmary Medical Center
P.O. Box 2144
Mobile, AL 36652
(205) 431-5559

Arizona

Sleep Disorders Center
Good Samaritan Medical Center
1111 East McDowell Road
Phoenix, AZ 85006
(602) 239-5815

Sleep Disorders Center
University of Arizona
1501 North Campbell Avenue
Tucson, AZ 85724
(602) 694-6112

Arkansas

Sleep Disorders Center
Arkansas Children's Center
800 Marshall Street
Little Rock, AR 72202–3591
(501) 370-1893

Sleep Disorders Center
Baptist Medical Center
9601 l-630, Exit 7
Little Rock, AR 72205–7299
(501) 227-1902

Sleep Disorders Diagnostic &
   Research Center
University of Arkansas for Medical
   Sciences
4301 West Markham, Slot 594
Little Rock, AR 72205
(501) 686-6300

California

WMCA Sleep Disorders Center
Western Medical Center-Anaheim
1101 South Anaheim Boulevard
Anaheim, CA 92805
(714) 491-1159

Sleep Disorders Center
Downey Community Hospital
11500 Brookshire Avenue
Downey, CA 90241
(213) 806-5280

Sleep Disorders Institute
St. Jude Hospital
   and Rehabilitation Center
101 East Valencia Mesa Drive
Fullerton, CA 92634
(714) 871-3280

Sleep Disorders Center
Scripps Clinic and Research
   Foundation
10666 North Torrey Pines Road
La Jolla, CA 92037
(619) 554-8087

The Hospital of the Good Samaritan
616 South Witmer Street
Los Angeles, CA 90017
(213) 977-2206

UCLA Sleep Disorders Clinic
Department of Neurology
Room 1184, RNRC
710 Westwood Plaza
Los Angeles, CA 90024
(213) 206-8005

North Valley Sleep Disorders Center
11550 Indian Hills Road, Suite 291
Mission Hills, CA 91345
(818) 898-4639

Sleep Disorders Center
Hoag Memorial Hospital
   Presbyterian
301 Newport Boulevard
Newport Beach, CA 92663
(714) 760-2070

Sleep Apnea Center
Merritt–Peralta Medical Center
450 30th Street
Oakland, CA 94609
(415) 451-4900, Ext. 2273

Sleep Disorders Center
U.C. Irvine Medical Center
101 City Drive South
Orange, CA 92668
(714) 634-5105

Sleep Disorders Center
Huntington Memorial Hospital
100 Congress Street
Pasadena, CA 91105
(818) 397-3061

Sleep Disorders Center
Pomona Valley Hospital Medical
  Center
1798 North Garey Avenue
Pomona, CA 91767
(714) 865-9135

Sleep Disorders Center
Sequoia Hospital
Whipple and Alameda
Redwood City, CA 94062
(415) 367-5137

Sutter Sleep Disorders Laboratory
Sutter Hospitals
52nd and F Streets
Sacramento, CA 95819
(916) 733-1070

San Diego Regional
  Sleep Disorders Center
Harbor View Medical Center
  and Hospital
120 Elm Street
San Diego, CA 92101
(619) 235-3176

Sleep Disorders Clinic
Stanford University Medical Center
Hoover Pavilion, Second Floor
211 Quarry Road, N2A
Stanford, CA 94305
(415) 723-6601

Southern California
  Sleep Apnea Center
Lombard Medical Group
2230 Lynn Road
Thousand Oaks, CA 91360
(805) 495-1066

Sleep Disorders Center
Torrance Memorial Hospital
3330 Lomita Boulevard
Torrance, CA 90509
(213) 517-4617

Sleep Disorders Center
Kaweah Delta District Hospital
400 West Mineral King Avenue
Visalia, CA 93291
(209) 625-7303

Pediatric Sleep Apnea Laboratory
Queen of the Valley Hospital
1115 South Sunset Avenue
West Covina, CA 91790
(818) 962-4011

Colorado

National Jewish Center for
  Immunology and Research
  Medicine
Cardio-Respiratory Sleep Disorders
  Center
1400 Jackson
Denver, CO 80206
(303) 398-1426

Sleep Disorders Center
University of Colorado Health
  Sciences Center
700 Delaware Street
Denver, CO 80204
(303) 592-7278

Connecticut

Sleep Disorders Center
The Griffin Hospital
130 Division Street
Derby, CT 06418
(203) 732-7560

New Haven Sleep Disorders Center
100 York Street
University Towers
New Haven, CT 06511
(203) 776-9578

District of Columbia

Sleep Disorders Center
Georgetown University Hospital
3800 Reservoir Road NW
Washington, DC 20007–2197
(202) 784-3610

Florida

Sleep Disorder Laboratory
Broward General Medical Center
1600 South Andrews Avenue
Fort Lauderdale, FL 33316
(305) 355-5534

Center for Sleep Disorder Breathing
St. Vincent's Medical Center
P.O. Box 2982
Jacksonville, FL 32203
(904) 387-7300, Ext. 8743

Sleep-Related Breathing
    Disorders Center
Baptist Medical Center
800 Prudential Drive
Jacksonville, FL 32207
(904) 393-2909

Sleep Disorders Center
Mt. Sinai Medical Center
4300 Alton Road
Miami Beach, FL 33140
(305) 674-2613

Georgia

Sleep Disorders Center
Northside Hospital
1000 Johnson Ferry Road
Atlanta, GA 30342
(404) 851-8135

Savannah Sleep Disorders Center
Saint Joseph's Hospital
P.O. Box 60129
Savannah, GA 31420–0129
(912) 927-5141

Hawaii

Sleep Disorders Center of the Pacific
Straub Clinic & Hospital
888 South King Street
Honolulu, HI 96813
(808) 522-4448

Illinois

Sleep Disorders Center
Rush–Presbyterian–St.Luke's
1753 West Congress Parkway
Chicago, IL 60612
(312) 942-5440

Sleep Disorders Center
University of Chicago
5841 South Maryland, Box 425
Chicago, IL 60637
(312) 702-0648

Center for Sleep-Related
    Breathing Disorders
Decatur Memorial Hospital
2300 North Edward
Decatur, IL 62526
(217) 877-8121, Ext. 5405

Sleep Disorders Center
Evanston Hospital
2650 Ridge Avenue
Evanston, IL 60201
(312) 492-4983

C. Duane Morgan Sleep
    Disorders Center
Methodist Medical Center of Illinois
221 Northeast Glen Oak
Peoria, IL 61636
(309) 672-4966

Carle Regional Sleep
  Disorders Center
602 West University
Urbana, IL 61801
(217) 337-3364

Indiana

Sleep Disorders Center
Winona Memorial Hospital
3232 North Meridian Street
Indianapolis, IN 46208
(317) 927-2100

Sleep/Wake Disorders Center
Community Hospitals Indianapolis
1500 North Ritter Avenue
Indianapolis, IN 46219
(317) 353-4275

Sleep Alertness Center
Lafayette Home Hospital
2400 South Street
Lafayette, IN 47903
(317) 447-6811

Iowa

Sleep Disorders Center
Mercy Hospital
West Central Park at Marquette
Davenport, IA 52804
(319) 383-1071

St. Luke's Sleep Disorders Center
  For Sleep-Related
  Breathing Disorders
1227 East Rusholme Street
Davenport, IA 52803
(319) 326-6740

Sleep Disorders Center
Iowa Methodist Medical Center
1200 Pleasant Street
Des Moines, IA 50309
(515) 283-5094

Kentucky

Sleep Disorders Center
St. Joseph's Hospital
One St. Joseph Drive
Lexington, KY 40504
(606) 278-3436, Ext. 1855

Sleep Disorders Center
Humana Hospital–Audubon
One Audubon Plaza Drive
Louisville, KY 40217
(502) 636-7459

Louisiana

Tulane Sleep Disorders Center
1415 Tulane Avenue
New Orleans, LA 70112
(504) 584-3592

LSU Sleep Disorders Center
Louisiana State University
  Medical Center
P.O. Box 33932
Shreveport, LA 71130–3932
(318) 674-5365

Maine

Sleep Laboratory
Maine Medical Center
22 Bramhall Street
Portland, ME 04102
(207) 871-2279

Maryland

The Johns Hopkins
  Sleep Disorders Center
Francis Scott Key Medical Center
Baltimore, MD 21224
(301) 550-0571

National Capital Sleep Center
4520 East West Highway
Number 406
Bethesda, MD 20814
(301) 656-9515

Massachusetts

Sleep Disorders Unit
Beth Israel Hospital
330 Brookline Avenue, KS430
Boston, MA 02215
(617) 735-3237

Michigan

Sleep/Wake Disorders Unit
VA Medical Center
Southfield and Outer Drive
Allen Park, MI 48101
(313) 562-6000, Ext. 3662

Sleep Disorders Center
University of Michigan Hospitals
1500 East Medical Center Drive
Med Inn C433, Box 0842
Ann Arbor, MI 48109–0115
(313) 936-9068

Sleep Disorders Center
Henry Ford Hospital
2799 West Grand Boulevard
Detroit, MI 48202
(313) 972-1800

Sleep Disorders Program
Ingham Medical Center
401 West Greenlawn Avenue
Lansing, MI 48910–2819
(517) 334-2510

Sleep Disorders Institute
Beaumont Hospital Medical Building
44199 Dequindre, Suite 403
Troy, MI 48098
(313) 54-SLEEP

Minnesota

Duluth Regional Sleep
   Disorders Center
St. Mary's Medical Center
407 East Third Street
Duluth, MN 55805
(218) 726-4692

Sleep Disorders Center
Abbott Northwestern Hospital
800 East 28th Street
   at Chicago Avenue
Minneapolis, MN 55407
(612) 863-3200

Sleep Disorders Center
Neurology Department
Hennepin County Medical Center
701 Park Avenue South
Minneapolis, MN 55415
(800) 343-6774

Sleep Disorders Center
Mayo Clinic
200 First Street SW
Rochester, MN 55905
(507) 286-8900

Sleep Disorders Center
Methodist Hospital
6500 Excelsior Boulevard
St. Louis Park, MN 55426
(612) 932-6083

Mississippi

Sleep Disorders Center
Memorial Hospital at Gulfport
P.O. Box 1810
Gulfport, MS 39501
(601) 865-3152 or (601) 865-3495

Sleep Disorders Center
University of Mississippi
   Medical Center
2500 North State Street
Jackson, MS 39216-4505
(601) 984-4820

Missouri

Sleep Disorders Center
Research Medical Center
2316 East Meyer Boulevard
Kansas City, MO 64132–1199
(816) 276-4222

Sleep Disorder Center
Deaconess Hospital
6150 Oakland Avenue
St. Louis, MO 63139
(314) 768-3100

Sleep Disorders Center
St. Louis University Medical Center
1221 South Grand Boulevard
St. Louis, MO 63104
(314) 577-8705

Sleep Disorders Center
L. E. Cox Medical Center
3801 South National Avenue
Springfield, MO 65807
(417) 885-6189

Nebraska

Sleep Disorders Center
Lutheran Medical Center
515 South 26th Street
Omaha, NE 68103
(402) 536-6352

New Hampshire

Sleep-Wake Disorders Center
Hampstead Hospital
East Road
Hampstead, NH 03841
(603) 329-5311, Ext. 240

Dartmouth-Hitchcock
  Sleep Disorders Center
Department of Psychiatry
Dartmouth Medical School
703 Remsen
Hanover, NH 03756
(603) 646-7534

New Jersey

Sleep Disorders Center
Newark Beth Israel Medical Center
201 Lyons Avenue
Newark, NJ 07112
(201) 926-7163

New York

Sleep-Wake Disorders Center
Montefiore Hospital
111 East 210th Street
Bronx, NY 10467
(212) 920-4841

Sleep Disorders Center
  of Western New York
Millard Fillmore Hospital
3 Gates Circle
Buffalo, NY 14209
(716) 884-9253

Sleep Disorders Center
Columbia–Presbyterian
  Medical Center
161 Fort Washington Avenue
New York, NY 10032
(212) 305-1860

Sleep Disorders Center
St. Mary's Hospital
89 Genesee Street
Rochester, NY 14611
(716) 464-3391

Sleep Disorders Center of Rochester
2110 Clinton Avenue South
Rochester, NY 14618
(716) 442-4141

Sleep Disorders Center
University Hospital
MR 120 A
Stony Brook, NY 11794–7139
(516) 444-2916

The Sleep Center
Community General Hospital
Broad Road
Syracuse, NY 13215
(315) 492-5877

Sleep-Wake Disorders Center
New York Hospital–Cornell
  Medical Center
21 Bloomingdale Road
White Plains, NY 10605
(914) 997-5751

North Carolina

Sleep Disorders Center
University Memorial Hospital
P.O. Box 560727
W. T. Harris Boulevard at U.S. 29
Charlotte, NC 28256
(704) 547-9556

North Dakota

Sleep Disorders Center
St. Luke's Hospital
720 Fourth Street North
Fargo, ND 58122
(701) 234-5673

Ohio

The Center for Research
  in Sleep Disorders
Affiliated with Mercy Hospital of
  Hamilton/Fairfield
1275 East Kemper Road
Cincinnati, OH 45246
(513) 671-3101

Sleep Disorders Center
Bethesda Oak Hospital
619 Oak Street
Cincinnati, OH 45206
(513) 569-6320

Sleep Disorders Center
Department of Neurology
Cleveland Clinic
9500 Euclid Avenue
Cleveland, OH 44106
(216) 444-2165

Sleep Disorders Treatment
  and Research
Ohio State University
473 West 12th Avenue
Columbus, OH 43210
(614) 293-8296

The Center for Sleep
  and Wake Disorders
Miami Valley Hospital
Suite G200
Thirty Apple Street
Dayton, OH 45409
(513) 220-2515

Northwest Ohio Sleep
  Disorders Center
The Toledo Hospital
2142 North Cove Boulevard
Toledo, OH 43606
(419) 471-5629

Sleep Disorders Center
St. Vincent Medical Center
2213 Cherry Street
Toledo, OH 43608–2691
(419) 321-4980

Oklahoma

Sleep Disorders Center
Presbyterian Hospital
Northeast 13th at Lincoln Boulevard
Oklahoma City, OK 73104
(405) 271-6312

Oregon

Pacific Northwest Sleep/Wake
  Disorders Program
  and Medical Center
Good Samaritan Hospital
1130 Northwest 22nd Avenue
Portland, OR 97210
(503) 229-8311

Sleep Disorders Center
Rogue Valley Medical Center
2825 Barnett Road
Medford, OR 97504
(503) 770-4320

Pennsylvania

Sleep Disorders Center
Jefferson Medical College
1015 Walnut Street, Third Floor
Philadelphia, PA 19107
(215) 928-6175

Sleep Disorders Center
The Medical College
  of Pennsylvania
3200 Henry Avenue
Philadelphia, PA 19129
(215) 842-4250

Sleep Evaluation Center
Western Psychiatric Institute
3811 O'Hara Street
Pittsburgh, PA 15213–2593
(412) 624-2246

Sleep Disorders Center
Department of Neurology
Crozer–Chester Medical Center
Upland, PA 19013
(215) 447-2689

South Carolina

Children's Sleep Disorders Center
Self Memorial Hospital
1325 Spring Street
Greenwood, SC 29646
(803) 227-4449 or (803) 227-4206

Sleep Disorders Center
Baptist Medical Center
Taylor at Marion Streets
Columbia, SC 29220
(803) 771-5847

South Dakota

Sleep Disorders Center
Sioux Valley Hospital
1100 South Euclid
Sioux Falls, SD 57117–5039
(605) 333-6302

Tennessee

Sleep Disorders Center
Fort Sanders Regional
  Medical Center
1901 West Clinch Avenue
Knoxville, TN 37916
(615) 541-1375

Sleep Disorders Center
St. Mary's Medical Center
Oak Hill Avenue
Knoxville, TN 37917
(615) 971-7529

Sleep Disorders Center
Baptist Memorial Hospital
899 Madison Avenue
Memphis, TN 38146
(901) 522-5704

Sleep Disorders Center
Saint Thomas Hospital
P.O. Box 380
Nashville, TN 37202
(615) 386-2068

Sleep Disorders Center
West Side Hospital
2221 Murphy Avenue
Nashville, TN 37203
(615) 329-6292

Texas

Sleep-Wake Disorders Center
Presbyterian Hospital
8200 Walnut Hill Lane
Dallas, TX 75231
(214) 696-8563

Sleep Disorders Center
Sun Towers Hospital
1801 North Oregon
El Paso, TX 79902
(915) 532-6281

Sleep Disorders Center
All Saints Episcopal Hospital
1400 Eighth Avenue
Fort Worth, TX 76104
(817) 927-6120

Sleep Disorders Center
Baylor College of Medicine
One Baylor Plaza
Houston, TX 77030
(713) 799-4886

Sleep Disorders Center
Sam Houston Memorial Hospital
8300 Waterbury
Suite 350
Houston, TX 77055
(713) 973-6483

Sleep Disorders Center
Scott and White Clinic
2401 South 31st Street
Temple, TX 76508
(817) 774-2554

Utah

Sleep Disorders Center
Utah Neurological Clinic
1055 North 300 West
Suite 400
Provo, UT 84604
(801) 379-7400

Intermountain Sleep Disorders
  Center
LDS Hospital
325 Eighth Avenue
Salt Lake City, UT 84143
(801) 321-3417

Virginia

Sleep Disorders Center
Eastern Virginia Medical School
Sentara Norfolk General Hospital
600 Gresham Drive
Norfolk, VA 23507
(804) 628-3322

Sleep Disorders Center
Medical College of Virginia
P.O. Box 710–MCV
Richmond, VA 23298
(804) 786-1993

Sleep Disorders Center
Community Hospital
  of Roanoke Valley
P.O. Box 12946
Roanoke, VA 24029
(703) 985-8435

Washington

Sleep Disorders Center
Providence Medical Center
500 17th Avenue, C-34008
Seattle, WA 98124
(206) 326-5366

Jeffrey C. Elmer, M.D.
Sleep Apnea Center
Sacred Heart Medical Center
West 101 Eighth Avenue, TAF-C9
Spokane, WA 99220–4045
(509) 455-3131

Wisconsin

Wisconsin Sleep Disorders Center
Gundersen Clinic, Ltd.
1836 South Avenue
La Crosse, WI 54601
(608) 782-7300

Milwaukee Regional
  Sleep Disorders Center
Columbia Hospital
2025 East Newport Avenue
Milwaukee, WI 53211
(414) 961-4650

Sleep/Wake Disorders Center
St. Mary's Hospital
2323 North Lake Drive
Milwaukee, WI 53201–0503
(414) 225-8032

Canada

Alberta

Sleep Disorders Clinic
Foothills Hospital
University of Calgary
1403 29th Street NW
Calgary, Alberta T2N 2T9
(403) 283-2669

Sleep Disorders Clinic
University of Alberta
I-134 Clinical Sciences Building
Edmonton, Alberta T6G 2G3
(403) 432-6567

British Columbia

Sleep Disorders Laboratory
University Hospital UBC Site
2211 Westbrook Mall
Vancouver, British Columbia
  V6T 2B5
(604) 228-7128

Sleep Laboratory
Royal Jubilee Hospital
1900 Fort Street
Victoria, British Columbia V8R 1J8
(604) 595-9200

Manitoba

Sleep Disorders Clinic
St. Boniface Hospital
409 Tache Avenue
Winnepeg, Manitoba R2H 2A6
(204) 237-2760

Ontario

Sleep Disorders Clinic
McMaster University
  Medical Center
1200 Main Street West
Hamilton, Ontario L8S 4J1
(416) 521-2100

Sleep Disorders Clinic
Ottawa General Hospital
501 Smyth Road
Ottawa, Ontario K1H 8L6
(613) 737-8155

Sleep Disorders Center
Sunnybrook Medical Center
2075 Bayview Avenue
Toronto, Ontario M4N 3M5
(416) 480-4693

Sleep Disorders Center of
  Metropolitan Toronto
537 Lawrence Avenue West
Toronto, Ontario M6A 1A3
(416) 785-1128

Sleep Disorders Clinic
St. Michael's Hospital
30 Bond Street
Toronto, Ontario M3J 1W8
(416) 864-5190

Sleep Disorders Clinic
Toronto Western Hospital
399 Bathurst Street
Toronto, Ontario M5T 2S8
(416) 368-2581

Sleep Laboratory
Hospital for Sick Children
555 University Avenue
Toronto, Ontario M5G 1X8
(416) 598-1500

Sleep Laboratory
Queen Elizabeth Hospital
550 University Avenue
Toronto, Ontario M5G 2A2
(416) 598-5111

Quebec

Sleep Disorders Clinic
Hospital du Sacre-Coeur
5400 Boulevard, Gouin Quest
Montreal, Quebec H4J 1C5
(514) 333-2692

Other International Centers

Argentina

Laboratorio de Estudio del Sueño y
   la Vigilia
Departmento de Neurofisiologia
   Clinica
Ayacucho 2166
1112 Buenos Aires
Argentina

Australia

Sleep Center
Department of Medicine
University of Sydney
Sydney
New South Wales 2006
Australia

Sleep Disorders Clinic
Department of Medicine
Royal Prince Alfred Hospital
Missenden Road
Camperdown
New South Wales 2050
Australia

Sleep Disorders Unit
Epworth Hospital
Erim Street
Richmond
Victoria 3121
Australia

Belgium

Laboratoire de Sommeill
Hospital Erasme
808 Route de Lennik
B-1070 Brussels
Belgium

Sleep-Wake Disorders Center
University Hospital of Antwerp
Wilrijkstraat 10
B-2520 Edegem
Belgium

Czechoslovakia

Department of Neurology
Charles University
Katerinska 30
12000 Prague 2
Czechoslovakia

France

Laboratoire d'Etude du Sommeil
Hopital de la Salpetriere
47 Boulevard de l'Hopital
F-75651 Paris Cedex 13
France

Laboratoire du Sommeil
C. H. U. Rangueil
1 Ave J. Pouilhes
31054 Toulouse
France

Service: Sommeil-Reve
Hopital Neurologique
39 Boulevard Pinel
69500 Bron
France

Unite des Troubles du Sommeil
Centre Gui de Chaulia
34059 Montpellier
France

Israel

Sleep Laboratory
Gutwirth Building
Technion-Israel Institute of
    Technology
Technion City
Haifa 32000
Israel

Sleep Research Institute
Sheba Medical Center-Tel Hashomer
Ben Yehuda Street 79
Herzlia 46498
Israel

Sleep-Wake Disorders Center at
    Loewenstein
P.O. Box 3
Raanana
Israel

Italy

Centro del Sonno
Universita di Milano
Instituto di Scienze Biomediche
Ospedale S. Raffaele
2132 Milano
Italy

Clinica delle Malattie
Nervose et Mentali
Universita di Bologna
Via Ugo Foscolo 7
40123 Bologna
Italy

Japan

Sleep Disorders Clinic
Department of Neuropsychiatry
Kurume University School of
    Medicine
67 Asahi-machi
Kurume
830
Japan

Sleep Disorders Clinic
Department of Neuropsychiatry
Osaka University Medical School
1-1-50 Fukushima
Osaka
533
Japan

Sleep Disorders Clinic
Department of Psychiatry
Tokyo University School of
    Medicine
7-3-1 Hongo, Bunkyo-ku
Tokyo
113
Japan

New Zealand

Sleep Disorders Clinic
Department of Neurophysiology
Auckland Hospital
Auckland
New Zealand

Sleep Disorders Clinic
Department of Otolaryngology
Christchurch Hospital
Christchurch
New Zealand

Norway

Sleep Laboratory
Akershus Central Hospital
Clinical Neurophysiology Section
1474 Nordbyhagen
Norway

Republic of South Africa

Sleep Disorders Clinic
Department of Internal Medicine
University of the Orange Free State
Bloemfontein 9300
Republic of South Africa

Sleep Disorders Clinic
University of Cape Town
Groote Schuur Hospital
Observatory
Cape 7925
Republic of South Africa

Scotland

Sleep Disorders Clinic
Department of Psychiatry
University of Edinburgh
Teviot Place
Edinburgh EH89AG
Scotland

U.S.S.R.

Sleep Disorders Center
First Moscow Medical Institute
Moscow

Sleep Disorders Associations, Organizations, and Support Groups

American Sleep Disorders
   Association
604 Second Street SW
Rochester, MN 55902
(507) 287-6006

American Sleep Disorders
   Foundation
112 Massachusetts Avenue
Arlington, MA 02174
(617) 648-8805

American Narcolepsy Association
P.O. Box 1187
San Carlos, CA 94070
(415) 591-7979

A.W.A.K.E.
(Alert, Well, And Keeping Energetic)
Health awareness and support
   groups for patients with sleep
   apnea. For information about a
   group in your area, contact:

A.W.A.K.E. Network
Pulmonary Sleep Evaluation
   Center
Presbyterian-University
   Hospital
DeSoto at O'Hara Streets
Pittsburgh, PA 15213
(412) 647-3464

The Better Sleep Council
333 Commerce Street
Alexandria, VA 22314
For the brochure:
   "A to ZZZZ Guide to Better
   Sleep,"
   write to:

   The Better Sleep Council
   P.O. Box 13
   Washington, DC 20044

Useful Terms Defined

Acidosis: Disturbance in acid-base balance; increased blood acidity.

Adenoidectomy: Surgical removal of the adenoids.

Adenoids: Spongy lymphoid tissue in the area behind the nose (nasopharynx).

Apnea: Cessation of breathing for 10 seconds or more.

Apnea Index: Calculation of the frequency of apnea.

Arrhythmia: Abnormal heart rhythm.

Atonia: Intense muscle relaxation.

Bradycardia: Slowing of the heart rate.

Cardiologist: Physician specializing in the diagnosis and treatment of heart disease.

Circadian rhythm: Biological rhythm of the alternating sleep-wake cycles in a 24-hour day.

Collapsible airway: Soft tissues in the upper respiratory tract lacking any rigid support.

Deviated septum: Deflection of the cartilage that creates the nasal partition, usually causing obstructed breathing.

Electrocardiography (EKG): Recording and measurement of electrical heart muscle activity.

Electroencephalography (EEG): Recording and measurement of brain waves.

Electromyography (EMG): Recording and measurement of electrical muscle activity.

Electro-oculography (EOG): Recording and measurement of eye-muscle movement.

Enuresis: Loss of bladder control, with bed-wetting, during sleep.

Hypercapnia: Elevated blood level of carbon dioxide.

Hypersomnolence: Excessive tiredness or sleepiness during waking hours.

Hypertension: Elevated blood pressure.

Hypopnea: Reduced airflow (at least 50 percent) through the nose and mouth for 10 seconds or more.

Hypotonia: Reduced muscle tone.

Hypoxemia: Reduced blood level of oxygen.

Insomnia: Difficulty in getting to sleep and staying asleep.

Micro-arousal: Brief awakening during sleep.

Muscle tone: Degree of muscle tension or relaxation.

Myocardium: Heart muscles.

Narcolepsy: Central nervous system condition causing excess drowsiness during waking hours.

Nasal continuous positive airway pressure (Nasal CPAP): Pump that generates a constant air pressure through the nose.

Nasal polyp: Soft swelling arising from the mucous membrane of the nose or sinuses.

Nasal polypectomy: Surgical removal of polyps.

Nasal septoplasty: Surgery to correct a deviated nasal septum.

Nasopharynx: Area behind the nasal cavity, also referred to as the postnasal space.

Neurologist: Physician specializing in the diagnosis and treatment of nervous system disease.

Nocturnal myoclonus: Excess leg-muscle movement during sleep.

Non-rapid eye movement sleep (NREM sleep): Phase of sleep in which rapid eye movements do not occur.

Otolaryngologist: Physician specializing in the diagnosis and treatment of ear, nose, and throat diseases.

Oximeter: Device to measure blood-oxygen saturation.

Parasomnias: Various medical conditions that cause abnormal behavior during sleep.

Polysomnogram: Recording to measure a variety of physiological functions during sleep.

Polysomnographer: Physician or scientist trained in the interpretation of data gathered by polysomnography.

Pulmonologist: Physician specializing in the diagnosis and treatment of lung diseases.

Rapid eye movement sleep (REM sleep): Phase of sleep denoted by rapid eye movements.

Respiratory disturbance index: Calculation of the frequency of apnea.

Sinuses: Air-containing spaces closely related to the nasal cavities.

Sinusitis: Infection or inflammation in the mucous membrane lining of the sinuses.

Sleep cycles: Stages of sleep denoted by changes in brain wave activity.

Sleep disorders center (sometimes called sleep laboratory): Diagnostic facility designed to study sleep-related medical conditions.

Sleep fragmentation: Interruption of the normal sleep cycle.

Strain gauge: Device for measuring expansion of the chest and abdomen during inspiration.

Syndrome: Group of related symptoms, for example, the sleep apnea syndrome.

Tachycardia: Increase in heart rate.

Thermistor: Temperature-sensitive device to record airflow through the nose and mouth.

Tonsil: Spongy lymphoid tissue mass on either side of the pharynx.

Tonsillectomy: Surgical removal of the tonsils.

Tracheostomy: Surgery to open the windpipe.

Turbinectomy: Surgery to reduce the tissues on the inside walls of the nose.

Upper respiratory tract: Air passages leading to the lungs; structures included here are the nose, sinuses, throat, and larynx.

Uvulopalatopharyngoplasty (UPPP): Surgery to enlarge the air passages in the back of the throat.

Vasomotor rhinitis: Condition produced by an imbalance in nasal blood circulation, resulting in chronic nasal congestion.

Additional Reading

Suggested Books on Sleep and Its Disorders

Boulware, Marcus H. *Snoring.* New Jersey: American Faculty Press, 1974.

Dement, William. *Some Must Watch While Some Must Sleep.* New York: Charles Scribner and Sons, 1972.

Fairbanks, David N. F., Shiro Fujita, and Takenosuke Ikematsu. *Snoring and Obstructive Sleep Apnea.* New York: Raven Press, 1987.

Guilleminault, Christian, and William Dement. *Sleep Apnea Syndromes.* New York: Alan R. Liss, 1978.

Hales, Dianne. *The Complete Book of Sleep.* Massachusetts: Addison-Wesley, 1981.

Linde, Shirley, and Louis M. Savary. *The Sleep Book.* New York: Harper and Rowe, 1974.

Mendelson, Wallace. *Human Sleep and Its Disorders.* New York: Plenum Press, 1977.

Moore-Ede, M., F. Sulzman, and C. Fuller. *The Clocks That Time Us.* Massachusetts: Harvard University Press, 1982.

Orr, William C., Kenneth Altshuler, and Monte Stahl. *Managing Sleep Complaints.* Chicago: Yearbook Medical Publishers, 1982.

Parkes, J. D. *Sleep and Its Disorders.* Philadelphia: W. B. Saunders, 1985.

Riley, Terrance. *Clinical Aspects of Sleep and Sleep Disturbance.* New York: Butterworths, 1985.

Rosenthal, Lois. *How To Stop Snoring.* Cincinnati: Writer's Digest Books, 1986.

Saunders, Nicholas A. *Sleep and Breathing.* New York: Dekker, 1984.

Williams, Robert L. *Sleep Disorders: Diagnosis and Treatment.* New York: Wiley, 1978.

Selected Papers from the Medical Literature

Bailey, B. J. "Problematic Snoring and Sleep Apnea: The Place for Surgery." *Archives of Otolaryngology,* 110, 1984, 491–492.

Becker, K., and J. Cummiskey. "Managing Sleep Apnea: What are Today's Options?" *The Journal of Respiratory Diseases,* June, 1985, 50–71.

Berry, R. B., and A. J. Block. "Positive Nasal Airway Pressure Eliminates Snoring As Well As Obstructive Sleep Apnea." *Chest,* 85, 1984, 15–20.

Block, A. J. "Is Snoring A Risk Factor?" *Chest,* 80, 1981, 525–526.

Bradley, T. G., and E. A. Phillipson. "Pathogenesis and Pathophysiology of the Obstructive Sleep Apnea Syndrome." *Medical Clinics of North America,* 69, 1985, 1169–1185.

Broomes, E. L. "New Thoughts On Snoring Prevention." *Journal of the National Medical Association,* 74, 1982, 1139–1140.

Champion, P. C. "The Management of Snoring." *Medical Journal of Australia,* 143, 1985, 337–338.

Fairbanks, D. N. "Effects of Nasal Surgery on Snoring." *Southern Medical Journal,* 78, 1985, 268–270.

———. "Snoring: Surgical vs. Nonsurgical Treatment." *Laryngoscope,* 94, 1984, 1188–1192.

Felstein, I. "Snoring: The Sufferer Who Doesn't Suffer." *Nursing Mirror*, 148, 1979, 42–43.

Fujita, S. "Uvulopalatopharyngoplasty For Sleep Apnea and Snoring." *Ear, Nose and Throat Journal*, 63, 1984, 227–235.

Ghoneim, M. M. "Mechanism of Snoring." *Journal of the American Medical Association*, 245, 1981, 1729.

Gluckman, J. L. "The Clinical Approach to Nasal Obstruction." *The Journal of Respiratory Diseases*, April, 1983, 13–29.

Goldstein, J. A. "Possible Therapy For Snoring." *Western Medical Journal*, 138, 1983, 270–273.

———. "Protriptyline For Snoring." *New England Medical Journal*, 308, 1983, 1602.

Guilleminault, C., et al. "Sleep Apnea in Eight Children." *Pediatrics*, 58, 1976, 23–30.

Issa, F. G., and C. E. Sullivan. "Alcohol, Snoring and Sleep Apnea." *Journal of Neurology, Neurosurgery and Psychiatry*, 45, 1982, 353–359.

Jennett, S. "Snoring and Its Treatment." *British Medical Journal*, 289, 1984, 335–336.

Loughlin, G. N. "Obstructive Sleep Apnea in Older Children." *The Journal of Respiratory Diseases*, Oct., 1982, 10–19.

Morton, R. P., et al. "Surgery for Snoring—What Constitutes A Cure?" *New Zealand Medical Journal*, 98, 1985, 352.

Norton, P. G., E. V. Dunn, and J. S. Height. "Snoring in Adults: Some Epidemiologic Aspects." *Canadian Medical Association Journal*, 128, 1983, 674–675.

Powell, N., et al. "Obstructive Sleep Apnea, Continuous Positive Airway Pressure and Surgery." *Otolaryngology—Head and Neck Surgery*, 99, 1988, 362–369.

Riley, R. W., N. Powell, and C. Guilleminault. "Current Concepts for Treating Obstructive Sleep Apnea." *Journal of Maxillofacial Surgery*, 45, 1987, 149–157.

Simmons, F. B., et al. "Snoring and Some Obstructive Sleep Apnea Can Be Cured by Oropharyngeal Surgery." *Archives of Otolaryngology*, 109, 1983, 503–507.

————. "A Surgical Treatment for Snoring and Obstructive Sleep Apnea." *Western Journal of Medicine*, 140, 1984, 43–46.

Strohl, K. P., B. Cherniack, and B. Gothe. "Physiologic Basis of Therapy for Sleep Apnea." *American Review of Respiratory Diseases*, 134, 1986, 791–802.

Sussman, D., et al. "The Pickwickian Syndrome With Hypertrophy of Tonsils." *Laryngoscope*, 85, 1975, 565–569.

Tirlapur, V. G. "Snoring as a Risk Factor for Hypertension and Angina." *Lancet*, 1, 1985, 1340.

Westbrook, P. R. "The Chronically Snoring Child: An Acoustic Annoyance or Cause for Concern? *Mayo Clinical Proceedings*, 58, 1983, 399.

Wilson, K., et al. "Snoring: An Acoustic Monitoring Technique." *Laryngoscope*, 95, 1985, 1174–1177.

Zwillich, C. "The Clinical Significance of Snoring." *Archives of Internal Medicine*, 139, 1979, 24.

Popular Magazine Articles on Snoring

"How Can George Stop Snoring?" *Ladies' Home Journal*, April, 1915, 32:54.

"Why We Snore." *Literary Digest*, 1924, 83:27.

Bilik, S. "About Why People Snore." *Hygeia*, 1946, 24:820.

Dugan, James. "Bedlam in the Boudoir." *Collier's*, 1947, 119:17.

"For Sonorous Sleepers." *Newsweek*, 1949, 33:46.

"Conquest of Snoring Claimed." *Science*, 1950, 58:359.

"A Cure for Snoring." *Scientific American*, 1951, 184:35.

"A Cure for Snoring." *Today's Health*, April, 1953, 31:6.

"Husband's Snore Claimed Sign of Affection." *Science Digest*, 1954, 35:29.

Fabricant, Noah. "Sound Facts About Snoring." *Today's Health*, 1958, 36:18.

Waggoner, Walter. "About Snoring." *New York Times Magazine,* Oct., 1960, 16:43.

"Can Snoring Be Cured?" *Good Housekeeping,* 1962, 155:137.

Van Buren, Abigail. "Is There a Snorer in the House?" *Reader's Digest,* 1966, 89:114.

Snider, A. "Putting a Stop to Snoring." *Science Digest,* 1972, 71:59.

"Help for Snorers." *Modern Maturity,* 1976, 19:15.

Cohen, Marcia. "Things That Go Z-Z-Z in the Night." *Ladies' Home Journal,* 1976, 93:56.

Buffington, P. "The Sounds of Sleep." *Saturday Evening Post,* 1981, 253:74.

"How to Get a Good Night's Sleep With A Man." *Glamour,* 1981, 79:146.

"Snore-Breakers." *Fifty Plus,* 1981, 21:26.

"Snoring Cure." *Omni,* 1981, 4:49.

"The Better Mouth Trap." *Weightwatchers,* 1982, 15:12.

Cox, James. "Snorers! Don't Despair! There Will Always be UPPP." *Smithsonian,* 1983, 14:174.

"A Snip for A Snorer." *Health,* 1983, 15:22.

Kiester, E. "A Little Night Music." *Fifty Plus,* 1984, 24:68.

Lustig, Bill. "How to Be A Better Bedmate." *Glamour,* 1984, 82:56.

"New Surgical Treatment for Snoring." *USA Today,* 1984, 112:11.

Pechter, Kerry. "Surprising Facts about Snoring and Health." *Prevention,* 1984, 36:26.

"Relief for Nocturnal Noisemakers." *Science,* 1984, 5:92.

"Snore Wars: Surgery for Snorers." *Readers Digest,* 1984, 124:26.

"Snoring." *Good Housekeeping,* 1984, 199:58.

Wasco, James M. D. "All About Snoring from A to Z-Z-Z's." *Woman's Day,* 1984, September 9.

"Can You Snooze If He Snores?" *Mademoiselle,* 1985, 91:50.

"Snoring and Angina: A Link?" *Prevention,* 1985, 37:7.

"Snoring, Not Just Annoying Habit, But A Call for Help." *Better Homes and Gardens,* 1985, 63:72.

Credits

Text

pages 1, 8

FROM THE BEST OF DEAR ABBY
The Best of Dear Abby, copyright 1981 by
Phillips/Van Buren. Reprinted with
permission of Andrews & McMeel. All
rights reserved.

page 42

From a 1984 study by David Fairbanks,
M.D., *The Laryngoscope*, 1984.94
1188.1192, 1986.

page 156

Song by David Frishberg.

Illustrations

pages xii–xiii, 7,
46, 49, 51, 125

Leslie Flis.

page 2

Fabricant, Noah. "Sound Facts about
Snoring." *Today's Health* (1958): 36:18.

page 3

Cartoon by Peter Steiner. With
permission. *Smithsonian* (1983): 14:174.

pages 4, 104, 114

Boulware, Marcus H. *Snoring*. New Jersey:
American Faculty Press, 1974.

page 7

Based on an illustration from *Hearing in
Children*, page 7, 3d edition, by Jerry L.
Northern, Ph.D. Baltimore: Williams &
Wilkins Co.

pages 12, 14, 18   Reprinted, with permission, of Reader's
                        Digest Association, Inc.—September 1966
                        issue.

pages 25–27,   Jack Crane.
29–31, 35–38, 47,
52, 78–79, 133–34,
136, 142–43,
145–47, 149–50,
152

page 43   *MAD* Magazine © 1963, 1968, 1975, and
                        1986 by E. C. Publications, Inc.

page 46   Adapted from material by Olsen, Kerry D.,
                        M.D. "The Nose and its Impact on
                        Snoring and Obstructive Sleep Apnea."
                        Snoring and Obstructive Sleep Apnea,
                        edited by Fairbanks, David N. F., et al.,
                        New York: Raven Press, 1987.

page 61   PEANUTS Characters: © 1966, 1971,
                        United Features Syndicate, Inc.

pages 88, 134, 136   Reproduced, by permission, from
                        Respironics, Inc.

pages 90–91   Loughlin, Gerald M., M.D. "Obstructive
                        Sleep Apnea in Older Children." *The
                        Journal of Respiratory Diseases* (October
                        1982).

pages 103, 105–08,   *Official Gazette,* Washington, D.C.: U.S.
110–11   Patent and Trademark Office (June 1914).

page 115   Courtesy of Emanuel Hospital and Health
                        Center, Portland, Oregon.

Index

Page references in *italic* indicate illustrations.